What Others are Saying About This Self-Care Program:

"It's hard to believe that such simple, easy to follow exercises could have such a tremendous effect! Spending several hours a day at a computer is no longer the tedious, painful task it used to be."

-B. Keener, Data Processor

"The exercises are a pain-free, gentle way to restore range of motion and strength that I have not had in years. They fit naturally into my daily routine."

-E. Yespelkis, Registered Nurse and Homemaker

"Buy This Book! I have suffered through eight months of daily and nightly pain from Carpal Tunnel Syndrome and many consultations with doctors and alternative health practitioners. Once I began regular use of these clearly defined exercises I became flexible and pain free. I have avoided surgery and returned to daily writing and needlework. Yeah!"

-J. Pool, Clinical Social Worker

"Before these exercises I couldn't write. Now I can! I am so happy that I found an effective alternative to surgery!"

-J. Haas, Mother and Homemaker

"The exercises were illustrated well and the instructions easy to follow."

-O. Brady, Computer Programmer

"I use these exercises whenever I develop tightness as a result of playing the piano. I feel immediate release and relief."

-K. Brown, Piano Instructor

"I have experienced a marked improvement in my progressive and painful Carpal Tunnel Syndrome symptoms. These simple but extremely effective exercises have eliminated the need for surgery."

-A. Wallace, Administrative Assistant

"I am happily back to needlepointing and piano playing once more!"

-L. Horowitz, Homemaker

"I practice the exercises twice a day. My Carpal Tunnel Syndrome symptoms are measurably improved."

-P. Shenian, Chemist

"I have certainly benefited from these exercises. I have much less pins and needles in my hands at night and almost no neck cramps."

-F. Statzell, Registered Nurse

"Using the exercises for pain and tension in my neck and shoulders has given me noticeably increased mobility. I found them easy to follow and the drawings especially helpful. Thank you!"

-A. Marquart, Administrative Assistant

"I have learned to pay attention to my body in new ways and using this new, heightened sensitivity, I have become aware of how I have been sitting, standing, sleeping, and breathing. The changes I have made through this program have kept my Carpal Tunnel Syndrome symptoms from returning."

-L. Lang, Computer Programmer

"These exercises are minor miracles! If the ABC's in school included this kind of stretching, we'd have a far healthier country!"

-H. Haven, House Doctor

"I experienced immediate relief using this exercise program. I could feel my hands and arms releasing years of tension. No "experts" could do this for me. My life is finally getting back in order."

- D. Gentile, Seamstress

"I found relief from pain with use of the exercises on a regular basis. The instructions are easy to understand and helpful as a reminder of how to do the exercises correctly."

-S. Bierker, Psychotherapist

CONQUERING CARPAL TUNNEL
Syndrome

and other

Repetitive Strain Injuries

A Self-Care Program

Sharon J. Butler

Illustrated by Jacqueline Entwistle Freeman

New Harbinger Publications
Oakland, CA

Design by Carriage House Designs, Villanova, PA
Illustrations by Jacqueline Entwistle Freeman

Published for the trade by New Harbinger
    Publications, 5674 Shattuck Avenue,
    Oakland, CA 94609

Special sales and marketing by Advanced Press,
    1708 Lancaster Ave., #321, Paoli, PA 19301

Printed on recycled paper

Library of Congress Catalog Number: 94-96893
ISBN 1-57224-039-3 Paperback

Distributed in the U.S.A. primarily by Publishers
Group West; in Canada by Raincoast Books; in
Great Britain by Airlift Book Company, Ltd.; in
South Africa by Real Books, Ltd.; in Australia by
Boobook; and in New Zealand by Tandem Press.

Printed in the United States of America

00   99

15   14   13   12   11   10   9   8   7

This book is dedicated to

Daniel Eldridge.

He was the first person

who told me I was a powerful woman.

I believed him

and it changed my life.

"Work with the hands is the

apprenticeship of honesty.

May the work of your hands

be a sign of gratitude and reverence

to the human condition."

-Gandhi

TABLE OF CONTENTS

ACKNOWLEDGMENTS

Fairy tales really do come true, but not without the help of special family and friends. My own list begins with my personal Fairy Godmother, Louise H. Moffitt. Without her support and assistance, this challenge would have been far more difficult. I have also been blessed with wonderful parents, Jack and Jean Butler, who have always believed in me and have given me everything I have needed to succeed. I am deeply indebted to Joseph Heller who is a constant source of inspiration and who taught me to see and appreciate the human body in a new and different way. Kathy Brown, Deborah Evans, Jacqueline Freeman, David Mintzer and Laura Partsch have also contributed significantly in the creation of this book. To these and all the countless others who have supported me with words of encouragement and confidence, I owe my deepest gratitude.

CONQUERING CARPAL TUNNEL SYNDROME

I developed Carpal Tunnel Syndrome in 1991. And like many of the people who will read this book, I too have suffered with numbness and tingling that awakened me at night, loss of strength in my hands and arms and the fear that I would have to change my career because the condition was robbing me of my ability to use my hands.

My career working with the human body began in 1984. Having searched out the most comprehensive and advanced training I could find for the study of muscles and connective tissues, I became certified in Hellerwork, and began a fascinating new career.

Hellerwork is, among other things, a bodywork technique used to restore the body to its normal state of alignment by the stretching and manipulation of connective tissues known as fascia. Fascia has very remarkable and unique properties which cause it to respond to various kinds of stress in ways that protect the body from injury. It is my understanding of the nature and function of fascia that has led to the development of the program outlined in this book.

When I first began experiencing symptoms of repetitive strain injury, I realized that those symptoms were related to changes occuring in the fascia of my hands, arms, shoulders, and neck. I used my bodywork skills to stretch these sore and restricted tissues and found significant relief almost immediately. Soon after, I developed a series of exercises which I could use at various times

MY STORY

of the day to help further restore my overworked hands and arms to their normal structural balance. Within days I was sleeping through the night without disturbance and was able to resume my normal work routine. I performed the exercises as needed to counteract the repetitive nature of my work.

Occasionally, I would feel symptoms recur. But performing the exercises always eliminated any discomfort. It was soon weeks and then months between any recurrence of symptoms. I was happy that I had an effective tool that could provide the relief I needed whenever the need arose.

I began offering my technique of bodywork and stretching exercise to other sufferers of Carpal Tunnel Syndrome and other repetitive strain injuries. My techniques worked just as well on them as on me.

Since 1991 I have been developing and assembling the series of exercises presented in this book. Practiced regularly, they can help relieve the symptoms of Carpal Tunnel Syndrome and repetitive strain injuries.

But the best use of this program is in the *prevention* of these life-changing disorders. I encourage you to begin the program if you are at risk for developing a repetitive strain injury. As the saying goes, "An ounce of prevention is worth a pound of cure."

INTRODUCTION

Carpal Tunnel Syndrome and other repetitive strain injuries of the hands and arms have become a modern-day menace in the workplace. Expensive, debilitating, and lifestyle threatening, they are changing the way workers and their employers are viewing jobs. Millions of dollars are spent yearly on medical treatments, ergonomic workstations, and worker's compensation benefits. Fortunately, much can be done to avoid the majority of these costs. Prevention is the key.

This book describes a self-care program for those at risk of developing Carpal Tunnel Syndrome and other repetitive strain injuries of the upper body, as well as for those who already suffer from these maladies. Some of the principles presented here are not new, while others might be considered daring or bold. However, they will prevent or reduce the effects of a repetitive strain injury if practiced properly.

It is my hope that this book will be an effective contribution to wellness in today's workplace, supporting greater productivity and profitability while enhancing the ability of each person to more fully enjoy his or her life and work.

Consult your physician before
beginning this or any other
exercise program.

SELF-CARE SUCCESS

The key to effective self-care is education. Once you become aware of how the soft tissues in your body are affected by posture and misuse and how this in turn can promote the occurrence of a repetitive strain injury, you will have some tools you can use to avoid these injuries.

In this section you will learn about your body and how it creates a repetitive strain injury, including Carpal Tunnel Syndrome. Read this section carefully. Understanding and using the concepts presented here will enhance your ability to effectively create a conditioning and prevention program that is best suited to your body's needs.

What is Connective Tissue?

Connective tissue is just what the name implies: tissue that connects. It is found everywhere in the body. Various types of connective tissues are blood, bone, tendons, and ligaments.

Connective tissue holds the body together, joining every part of the body with every other part. As the old song goes, the thigh bone really is connected to the hip bone. When considering the body in terms of the connective tissue, the big toe is also connected to the shoulder and the connective tissue that wraps the calf muscle is connected to the pericardium that wraps the heart.

The Unique Qualities of Connective Tissue

There is no beginning and no end to the connective tissue in the body. Everything blends into and becomes a part of everything else. Sometimes the tissue is superficial, perhaps just beneath the surface of the skin. Then it may go deeper, permeating through a muscle, becoming tendon and then blending into and becoming part of bone.

It is this unusual quality of connective tissue that can cause the perplexing array of symptoms so often experienced by persons suffering from an injury. Have you ever had a stiff neck? Did you notice that over a period of time, the pain seems to "travel," often extending down your back or out to your shoulder? The reason this happens is because in addition to connective tissue connecting everything to everything, it also acts as a transmitter. The strain of the original injury often is transmitted through the connective tissue to another area of the body.

Soon, what starts out as a stiff neck develops into a stiff neck-shoulder, or a stiff neck-back.

It is these interesting qualities of connective tissue that contribute greatly to the complexity of symptoms seen in repetitive strain injuries or Carpal Tunnel Syndrome. In any repetitive strain injury, whether it is a wrist problem caused by typing at a computer keyboard or a rotator cuff injury sustained by a major league baseball pitcher, the injury is rarely limited to the site of the pain. Each injury that involves connective tissue extends far beyond the original site of the injury. And for these injuries to heal effectively, all contributing factors and all affected areas of the body must be addressed. Connective tissue must be released wherever it has been strained.

What is Fascia?

Tendons and ligaments are each a type of connective tissue known as fascia. "Fascia" is a web-like form of connective tissue that holds tissue in suspension. Certain types of fascia known as myofascia permeate through muscle, first wrapping individual muscle fibers, then bundles of muscle fibers, then bundles of bundles, and finally, the entire muscle structure. Where the muscle fibers end, the myofascia that has been wrapping all of those fibers continues, becoming the tendon. Tendon actually blends into bone, becoming part of it. With a tensile strength greater than that of steel, fascia is an extremely durable component of the body.

Fascia Throughout the Body

Fascia also wraps and connects other parts of the body. When it wraps bone, fascia is called periosteum. It wraps blood vessels and nerve fibers, holding them in suspension, allowing them to "float" in a sea of muscle. Fascia, in the form of ligaments, suspends organs in their proper place. Fascia is everywhere.

When we move, muscle fibers contract, causing the fascia that wraps the muscle tissue to pull on its attached ends, the tendons. Since the tendons are connected to bone, they cause the bone to move.

Fascia and Movement

Fascia is not only closely related to the contraction of muscle tissue, but also to its release, or lengthening. For movement to happen, muscles on one side of a joint (the *agonists*) contract, causing the tendon to pull on the bone, encouraging movement. But for that movement to happen, muscles and connective tissue on the other side of the joint (the *antagonists*) have to release. The result is a constant "give and take," or contraction and lengthening. It is the quality of the coordination of this contraction versus lengthening process that helps determine the quality of movement - the strength, fluidity, and range of motion of the various parts of the body. When the contraction is strong and the corresponding release is unimpeded and fluid, the most effortless movement occurs. Joints move easily and gracefully. The body feels young and light.

So what causes the deterioration of movement? What makes it hard to use a part of the body without pain or discomfort?

Fascia's Response to Injury

Fascia is amazing stuff. It is part of the body's natural protection system, one of the body's best defenses against injury.

Fascia is endowed with an unusual property that enables it to be so helpful. It is capable of changing chemically, becoming sticky or dense when it is subjected to stress or injury.

Let's consider, for example, that you are rear-ended in a car accident. At the very moment of impact, the fascia in your neck senses that your neck is in peril, that it is in the process of receiving a whiplash injury. In an effort to save the spinal cord from harm, the fascia instantly becomes more solid and the fibers that make up the fascia become more densely packed. This, in effect, creates a sort of spontaneous, protective neck brace. And it all happens in the blink of an eye.

But, the fascia which created that spontaneous neck brace is not just connected to the muscles of your neck. It is also connected to your back, shoulders, chest, head, jaw, and hip. It is connected to everything in your body!

Any time a strain occurs in the body, the fascia responds by going through a chemical change. Such strains can take many forms. Any quick, forceful injury, such as the whiplash mentioned above, is cause for change in the fascia. Even bumping into the edge of a desk can have some effect on the fascia in the body.

Fascia and Scar Tissue

Another type of strain to the fascia is surgery or other types of wounds. In this case, the fascia is actually severed. In an effort to reconnect so that it can fulfill its bodily function, the fascia quickly forms scar tissue.

Scar tissue creates an interesting impact on the body. To better understand this impact, consider the qualities of a knitted sweater as an example.

A knitted sweater has lots of give and stretch in the fabric. It can stretch in all directions to a relatively equal degree. Imagine that the sweater tears. If the area around the tear is pulled, the sweater unravels and the hole in the sweater becomes larger. When it is repaired and the hole stitched shut, we can try to stretch the sweater in all directions. But now we find that there are new limits. The stretching stops at the point where the hole in the sweater was stitched closed. As a matter of fact, there are very few directions the sweater can be stretched without being affected by the stitched-up hole.

Scar tissue impacts the body in ways similar to the patched hole in the sweater. The ability of the body to stretch easily in all directions, or for a group of muscles to lengthen as the opposing group is contracted, is greatly affected by the presence of scar tissue, much like the repaired hole in the sweater. And once scar tissue is present, it can be its own source of strain, causing the fascia to solidify across broader sections of the body.

The Impact of Gravity

Gravity can also be a source of strain to fascia. Gravity is a force field that can either support the body structure or can lead to its deterioration. With good posture, natural body alignment is supported by gravity; with poor posture, gravity pulls down on whatever is out of alignment, such as a forward head, slumped shoulders, or a curved back. Such imbalance leads to the further inevitable decline of posture including pinched nerve fibers, herniated disks, and joints that do not move efficiently.

When gravity and poor posture begin to adversely affect the body, nothing moves as well as in the past. So how does the body protect itself from the constant onslaught of gravitational forces? Fascia comes to the rescue! The body needs more support in the face of all this downward pulling and strain. Fascia perceives the strain and begins to change. Some of the fascia becomes tough and fibrous, more like tendonous tissue. Other fascia becomes sticky, causing muscles that are next to one another to stick together, offering each other some measure of support.

The problem is that muscles must slide across one another as they contract and lengthen in order to get the body's work done. If they are stuck together, they cannot slide independently. They end up pulling each other along as they move. This makes the body feel heavy and movement becomes more strained and difficult. This, in turn, creates more strain on the fascia, resulting in greater restriction. Soon, whole sections of the body feel tight, weak, and strained. Because of poor posture and gravity, the cycle of deterioration continues and we feel old before our time.

The Human Body is Designed for Movement

The human body is designed for movement. Much of that movement, such as walking, is repetitive in nature. Under normal conditions, the repetitive nature of ordinary movement causes no problems. As a matter of fact, movement helps keep the fascia loose, fluid, and nonbinding. But when repetitive movement is combined with some other form of strain to the fascia such as poor posture or previous injury, then the repetitive nature of the movement takes on a limiting quality.

When fascia is subjected to repetitive movement at the same time it is being subjected to strain from injury or gravitational forces, the fascia will respond by protecting the body. It will tighten up and begin sticking muscle to muscle, or muscle to nerve, or nerve to ligament, and so on. The fascia does not respond so much to the repetitive nature of the movement as it does to other tissue-related strains in combination with the repetitive movement.

There's yet another problem. Once fascia becomes tight or stuck it cannot return to its former loose and fluid state without some form of intervention. The lifetime accumulation of a little tightness here and a little pulling there is what some people come to believe is the inevitable physical decline of aging.

Restoring Fascia to a More Normal State

Fascia supports us when we have been injured or have experienced other stresses or trauma in our bodies. Once the usefulness of this support is over, fascia must be restored to its normal loose state, allowing us to move again without strain or limitation. How do we accomplish this?

Stretching is an efficient way of restoring fascia to its normal, nonbinding state. Performed carefully and gently, stretching is a means of changing fascial tissues that is accessible to everyone.

Fascia is indeed amazing stuff. When we are injured or brought into a state of imbalance, fascia helps support us so that we do not end up in a rumpled heap on the floor. When the injury has healed, fascia can then be restored to balance and freedom of movement through simple stretching.

What are Repetitive Strain Injuries?

Repetitive strain injuries can occur in many different areas of the body. They are a result of repetitious movement of one or more parts of the body in combination with other forms of structural or fascial strain.

There are many forms of repetitive strain injury. Common examples include tennis elbow, knee problems in runners, and Carpal Tunnel Syndrome.

Repetitive movements, in and of themselves, are not the cause of repetitive strain injuries. Repetitive strain injuries are as much related to previous injury histories, posture or other traumas as they are to the repetitive nature of the movements we perform. They are also related to the strain we subject our bodies to while we are in the act of performing repetitive movement.

Let's consider two examples. Two people, A and B, work side by side as copywriters for a newspaper. Both people have symptoms of a repetitive strain injury: sore necks, aching shoulders, elbow pain, and numbness in the fingers. Same symptoms, same job. But here is where the similarities end.

Person A broke his arm when he was seven years old. Strain in the fascia of his arm, which was the result of the break and wearing a cast for several weeks, was never adequately released after the cast came off. His current symptoms of a repetitive strain injury may stem from those early days. The tissue that changed to a denser state long ago may still be affecting him today.

Person B has poor posture when sitting at her desk. The fascia in her body is strained by structural stress, creating opportunities for nerves to be pinched, breathing to be limited and gravity to pull down on the body in an unbalanced way.

Each person faces a unique challenge in overcoming their current symptoms. The person with the previously broken arm must find and stretch tissue that became stuck and rigid over many years. The second person has a different challenge to face. In addition to learning how to restore stressed fascial tissues to their normal state through stretching, she must be willing to learn new ways to use her body while seated at her desk. She must create new postural habits that support her body more effectively. In addition to stretching the tissue that has become tight, good workplace ergonomics will help overcome her problem.

Both people in these examples have an excellent chance of restoring their bodies to an optimum level of performance. It is not necessary that they continue to suffer with a repetitive strain injury. Through awareness and stretching they can regain a more youthful, unrestricted, and comfortable body.

What is Carpal Tunnel Syndrome?

Carpal Tunnel Syndrome is a type of repetitive strain injury.

The carpal tunnel is an area created by the configuration of the wrist bones. The bones of the wrist come together in the shape of a shallow valley. Passing through this shallow valley of bone are nine tendons. These tendons begin in muscles located in the forearms that help create the movement of the fingers. The median nerve, which brings feeling to the thumb, index, middle, and half of the ring finger, also passes through the carpal tunnel. Capping the carpal tunnel is a tough strap of ligament called the flexor retinaculum. With all of these bones, tendons, and nerves coming together in this manner, the carpal tunnel is a very crowded area.

As the fingers move, the tendons controlling that movement glide back and forth under the flexor retinaculum. If this area becomes irritated, the tendons can swell, squeezing the median nerve as they pass through the carpal tunnel.

Many sufferers of Carpal Tunnel Syndrome experience a considerable amount of discomfort in the forearm, upper arm, armpit, shoulder, and neck. Common symptoms include weakness, aching, burning, limited range of motion, numbness, and tingling. All of these symptoms can be caused by restriction of the fascia of the upper body. Weakness, aching, and limited range of motion are often caused by restriction in the fascia as it permeates through muscle tissue. Burning, numbness, and tingling can be caused when the fascia covering nerve tissue becomes stressed.

Specially designed stretching exercises can result in a very high degree of relief for sufferers of Carpal Tunnel Syndrome as well as other repetitive strain injuries. The charts found in this book are designed to guide you in determining which areas are affected by repetitive strain. By practicing the exercises suggested for your symptoms, you can begin the process of restoring your body to its normal, comfortable and fully functional state.

What is the Stretch Point?

Many of the exercises in this program refer to something called the Stretch Point. *The Stretch Point is the secret of success for this program.* If you can master the concept of the Stretch Point, you will achieve the best and quickest relief from your symptoms.

When most people think about stretching, they believe it should be approached with the same energy and intensity they apply to their regular exercise regimen. To them, hard and fast is the way to stretch. That good, hard-stretching "burn" is the desired sensation. But stretching in this manner is similar to trying to stretch a cold block of modeling clay. It takes a lot of energy and little gets done.

SELF-CARE SUCCESS

This approach *will not work* for Carpal Tunnel Syndrome and other repetitive strain injuries. Why? Symptoms of Carpal Tunnel Syndrome and repetitive strain injuries indicate that soft tissues in your hands, arms, shoulders, and neck, particularly the fascia, have undergone damaging changes. They are stressed and not capable of functioning like normal tissues. In order to be healed, these tissues require a softer, slower, gentler approach to stretching. This softer type of stretching is similar to trying to lengthen an inexpensive piece of plastic wrap without tearing it.

Imagine how a tiny stretch would feel to a damaged or sore muscle. If overworked tissue is asked to make a tiny change, it can do so quite easily. However, if you ask overworked tissue to make a big, dramatic change, it is already too sore or fatigued to be successful. All you will experience is more soreness, more fatigue. Be kind and gentle to your hurting muscles and connective tissues and they will be restored to health and normal function in the shortest possible time.

Achieving Self-Care with this Program

Here is how the Stretch Point can help you achieve true self-care with this program. The Stretch Point is the very beginning, the first hint of a stretch. Sometimes, there is no stretch sensation when you reach the Stretch Point, only a slight drag or resistance to the movement as you position your body for each exercise. If you hold your position at this point you will feel the Stretch Point sensation slowly develop, then fade as the tissue releases. With this release comes change, the kind of change that with continued practice leads to the restoration of your body to a more normal, pain-free state.

It takes a little practice to feel the Stretch Point properly. For many people it will be the first time they have really paid attention to the sensations they feel in their body. A simple way to feel the sensations more easily is to close your eyes as you practice each exercise. This helps eliminate visual distractions and helps you focus on the sensations you are feeling with the exercise.

So what should the Stretch Point feel like? Usually the Stretch Point will feel like a *tiny* stretch. The Stretch Point can also feel like a tiny aching sensation, usually occurring in the deeper muscles. This tiny sensation indicates that you are stretching softly enough to achieve the best and quickest results. You can also tell that you are stretching softly enough if you notice that the stretching or aching sensation disappears completely within ten to fifteen seconds. After you have felt the Release you can go on to the next tiny Stretch Point, or move on to the next exercise in your program.

What Should the Stretch Point Feel Like?

"Am I stretching properly or not?" This is a commonly asked question, and finding the answer requires a bit of experimentation. Begin the desired stretch and go to the point where you feel you are creating a Stretch Point. Close your eyes and try to feel the sensations

Proper Stretching Technique

of the stretch in as much detail as possible. Now decrease the stretch a tiny bit. Do you still feel a sensation of stretching? If you do, the first position was too hard a stretch and you were probably exceeding the Stretch Point. Repeat this process until all sense of stretching disappears. Return to the last position you were in where a Stretch Point could be felt. This will be a tiny sensation, quite comfortable, but with a sense that you are asking the tissue to change in a very gentle way. Congratulations! You have now found the correct Stretch Point. You should feel the stretch sensation completely disappear within ten to fifteen seconds. The next time you try to find the Stretch Point, you will be able to stretch farther because the release of the first Stretch Point has created more length in the tissue. You are on the way to restoring full function and health to your shortened and overworked tissues.

Here are a few more interesting points to consider when working with the Stretch Point. Muscles and fascia run throughout the body in many layers. These tissues will undergo changes according to the type of movement asked of them. It is conceivable that tissue in one area may not be restricted but the tissue immediately next to it is tighter and less able to move and stretch. When you find and release the Stretch Point in the less restricted tissue, the release may be immediately followed by a stronger stretching sensation because you have now accessed the tighter tissue. If you have this experience, simply reduce the stretch until you feel only the tiny Stretch Point in this tighter tissue. You will then be releasing the tighter tissue in the safest, most comfortable, and most permanent way.

The Cumulative Effect of Stretching

Working with stretching exercises using *tiny* Stretch Points has a cumulative effect. Consistently using the Stretch Point in the correct manner actually accelerates results and helps maintain these results over a more extended period. With practice, you should begin to notice that you can gradually stretch farther before finding the Stretch Point compared to the previous session. This is a sure sign that you are effectively and correctly using the Stretch Point. Congratulations! Keep up the good work!

What is the Release?

Almost every exercise in this book asks you to "wait for the Release." Why is this important?

The Release is your body's signal telling you that tight and restricted tissue has been changed. Each time you reach a Stretch Point, tight muscles are being asked to lengthen beyond their current capacity. The Release indicates that the stretching fascia and muscles have let go and are now actually longer in their relaxed state. The Release also tells you that you are making progress. Short and tight muscles are becoming longer and more fluid. They will feel stronger and have a higher level of endurance.

When you are correctly using the Stretch Point, you will feel a tiny stretching or aching sensation in your muscles. Sometimes the Release happens gradually, with a slow and gradual lessening of the sensation. At other times, the Release can happen quickly. When the Release occurs, the Stretch Point disappears completely and the muscle softens and lengthens.

It should take only ten to fifteen seconds to achieve a Release. If you find it takes longer for you, you are probably stretching too hard. Ease up on the stretch and notice how much smaller the Stretch Point feels in this new position. Once you experience the Release, you can go on to the next exercise.

How Often Should I Stretch?

Stretching is unique for each individual. Your stretching program may be different from someone who has similar symptoms. Your body's range of motion, the sensations you feel when stretching, and the stretches that are appropriate for your special needs are yours alone. Likewise, how often you stretch should be geared to the unique qualities of your connective tissue.

In trying to determine how often to stretch, it is helpful to think about a bank account. Imagine that when your fascia is injured by repetitive strain, your body is like a bank account that is overdrawn. Your muscles and connective tissues have worked beyond their capacity. They are more than fatigued and need more help than simple resting.

When you stretch, it's like adding funds back into your body's overdrawn bank account. If you stretch too hard, your body does not regain much of its working capacity and you add only $5.00 worth of healing back into your account. If you stretch properly, you deposit as much as $100.00 worth of healing into your account.

If you have injured tissues that are like an overdrawn bank account, it makes sense to add as many funds back into the account as possible before you start withdrawing funds in the form of more repetitive activities. It is important to practice your stretches properly. Doing so will replenish your account in the shortest amount of time.

The object of this self-care program is not only to get your body out of its overdrawn state but also to add enough funds back into your body's account so you can do just about any activity and not suffer further injury. Realize, however, that each physical activity you choose to do comes at a cost. Funds are withdrawn back out of the account each time you type, grasp, lift, write, and so on.

Consider the case of a person employed as an assembler. She has been on the job for several years and in the last 6 months, her hands have begun to hurt. What started as a minor ache that would go away with a little hand shaking has now turned into an unrelenting deep ache with occasional numbness. Her body's account is about $500.00 overdrawn. She selects a series of exercises from this program and practices them faithfully and carefully. Within one week, she is so much better that her hands no longer hurt constantly; she experiences intermittent problems only. At this point, her body is no longer overdrawn - her bank account is at about the $0.00 point.

The next day she goes back to work, performing her usual job activities that ordinarily contribute to her symptoms. By the end of the day her hands hurt again. Why? Every repetitive activity comes at a cost to the body. She has withdrawn further funds out of her body's healing account and is back into a negative balance.

The solution for repetitive strain injuries is to build up your body's healing account to the point where there is a surplus of funds in the account and then to maintain the account at that level. Every time you strain your tissues through work or leisure activities, funds are withdrawn from your account. If you started your day with $250.00 worth of funds in your account, and the day's activities cost you $150.00, you would most likely get through the entire day with no further symptoms of repetitive strain. If you do not replenish the account by stretching at the end of your day, restoring the account back to its $250.00 level, you will start the next day with an account worth $100.00. If the next day's activities cost you another $150.00 in healing funds, you will again be overdrawn. You most likely will begin to feel some symptoms return because you have again overdrawn your account.

Only you can determine how much your account is overdrawn. Only you can tell how much each exercise, practiced properly, is adding back into your account. And only you can tell when you have enough of a surplus in your account that you can do any activity without overdrawing your account all over again. You can tell all these things through experience and practice. Each time you practice a stretch, think about how your tissues feel as they change. Do you feel a full release? Do you get the sense that other areas need release? Do you practice proper posture when sitting or standing? How much tightness returns when you go through your normal day?

It is possible to restore your body to a state in which you can do all the things you want to do without pain, discomfort, or further damage. Practice your stretches carefully, thoughtfully, and consistently. You will soon be on the road to recovery and able to look forward to a pain-free future.

A Good Chair...

- ### Has adjustable seat height.

  The seat should be raised so the knees are level with or slightly lower than the hips and the feet are flat on the floor.

- ### Has adjustable arm rests.

  The arm rests should be positioned about one-half inch lower than the forearm and should not be used for constant support. Using the armrests encourages slouching and can cause shrugging in the shoulders. Even a slight shrugging in the shoulders will cause a build-up of stress in the neck, shoulders, and upper back.

- ### Has a seatback that can be locked in an upright position.

  Leaning back in the chair, even a little bit, causes the head to be positioned forward of the torso, unsupported by the shoulders. This leads to strain in the chest, neck, shoulders, and upper back.

Sitting is an activity that we spend a significant amount of time doing every day. Learning to sit properly and comfortably is very important when learning to avoid repetitive strain injuries.

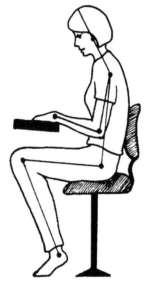

This person's sitting posture encourages muscular strain. Her head is forward of her torso and unsupported over her shoulders. This allows gravity to pull her head down. Muscles at the back of her neck must fight gravity constantly, fatiguing them. Her chest is depressed, reducing the fullness of her breath. Her elbows are forward of her torso and below the level of her desk. This causes her bicep and tricep muscles additional strain at the elbow. Her lower back is rounded, creating pain and encouraging her slumped posture. No wonder she feels tired and achy at the end of her day!

This person's body is well supported by gravity. Just like a straight stack of child's blocks, each segment sits squarely on the segment below it, providing effortless support. Her chest is open, allowing for full, complete breaths which will help sustain her energy for the day. Her lower back is aligned in its natural curve which minimizes strain. Her work is pulled close to the front of her body thus allowing her upper arms to hang straight down from shoulder to elbow. This eliminates tension at the shoulder, upper chest, and back. She appears more energetic and alert.

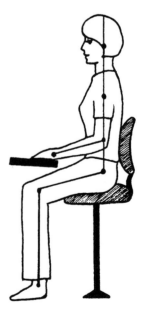

CHARTS

There are three sets of charts in this section designed to offer you assistance in setting up the stretching program best suited to your body's needs. They are:

• WHICH EXERCISES SHOULD I DO?

Use these charts if you already have symptoms of a repetitive strain injury. Find the chart which highlights the area of your body where you experience symptoms. Pick the section of the chart which most closely describes the qualities of your symptoms and proceed to the exercises suggested.

• PREVENTION BY PROFESSION

Use these charts if you currently experience only occasional or infrequent symptoms of repetitive strain injuries. Find the chart listing your profession and follow the exercise recommendations listed.

• TROUBLESHOOTING

Use these charts if you feel you are not getting the results you want from the exercises you have chosen. You may be able to get new ideas or awarenesses from the suggestions contained in these charts.

Please Note:
If, after consulting the charts in this section, you still cannot achieve the results you would like from the suggested exercises, reread the "Self-Care Success" section beginning on page 1. You may also find exercises more tailored to your unique needs by carefully reviewing all the exercises in the exercise sections. Each one lists the area of the body it is designed to help.

PROBLEM AREA	SYMPTOMS	EXERCISES	PAGE
NECK	Tight Stiff	Upper Body #1	52
		Upper Body #2	57
		Upper Body #3	58
		Upper Body #4	60
	Decreased Range of Motion	Upper Body #1	52
		Upper Body #4	60
		Upper Body #6	66
SHOULDERS	Tired Aching	Upper Body #3	58
		Upper Body #4	60
		Upper Body #7	70
	Tight	Upper Body #3	58
		Upper Body #7	70
		Upper Body #9	74
		Upper Body #13	84
	Decreased Range of Motion	Upper Body #10	76
		Upper Body #13	84
		Upper Body #14	86
		Upper Body #15	88

WHICH EXERCISES SHOULD I DO?

PROBLEM AREA	SYMPTOMS	EXERCISES	PAGE
• UPPER BACK •	Tight Restricted	Upper Body #3	58
		Upper Body #7	70
		Upper Body #10	76
	Rounded	Upper Body #7	70
		Upper Body #14	86
		Upper Body #15	88
	Pain Between Shoulder Blades	Upper Body #2	57
		Upper Body #5	62
		Upper Body #6	66
		Upper Body #16	90
• CHEST •	Tight	Upper Body #4	60
		Upper Body #10	76
		Upper Body #12	82
		Upper Body #15	88
	Slumped	Upper Body #7	70
		Upper Body #9	74
		Upper Body #14	86
		Upper Body #15	88

PROBLEM AREA	SYMPTOMS	EXERCISES	PAGE
• UPPER ARM •	Tight Aching	Upper Body #4	60
		Upper Body #8	72
		Upper Body #9	74
		Upper Body #15	88
	Weak Tired	Upper Body #10	76
		Upper Body #13	84
		Upper Body #16	90
• ARMPIT •	Tight	Upper Body #8	72
		Upper Body #9	74
		Upper Body #11	80
		Upper Body #14	86
	Decreased Range of Motion	Upper Body #10	76
		Upper Body #13	84
		Upper Body #14	86
		Upper Body #15	88

WHICH EXERCISES SHOULD I DO?

PROBLEM AREA	SYMPTOMS	EXERCISES	PAGE
• OUTER FOREARM •	Weak Tired	Forearms #2	96
		Wrists #10	124
		Fingers #6	137
	Aching Painful	Forearms #1	94
		Forearms #2	96
		Wrists #9	122
		Wrists #10	124
• INNER FOREARM •	Sore Aching	Forearms #1	94
		Forearms #3	98
		Wrists #3	110
		Wrists #8	121
	Loss of Strength	Forearms #3	98
		Forearms #4	101
		Wrists #8	121
		Fingers #5	135
	Numb Tingling	Wrists #4	112
		Wrists #5	116

WHICH EXERCISES SHOULD I DO?

PROBLEM AREA	SYMPTOMS	EXERCISES	PAGE
ELBOWS	Painful Sore	Upper Body #15	88
		Forearms #2	96
		Forearms #3	98
	Nerve Discomfort	Forearms #1	94
		Forearms #3	98
		Forearms #5	102
WRISTS	Sore Aching	Wrists #1	106
		Wrists #3	110
		Wrists #4	112
		Wrists #5	116
	Decreased Range of Motion	Wrists #1	106
		Wrists #2	108
		Wrists #6	118
		Wrists #7	120

WHICH EXERCISES SHOULD I DO?

PROBLEM AREA	SYMPTOMS	EXERCISES	PAGE
• PALM •	Tight Restricted	Fingers #1	128
		Thumbs #4	146
	Sore Aching	Fingers #1	128
		Fingers #3	133
	Numb Tingling	Upper Body #1	52
		Upper Body #4	60
		Upper Body #14	86
		Forearms #3	98
		Wrists #5	116
		Fingers #1	128
• THUMBS •	Aching Sore	Thumbs #5	148
		Thumbs #6	150
		Thumbs #7	152
	Decreased Range of Motion	Thumbs #3	144
		Thumbs #4	146
		Thumbs #7	152
	Lack of Strength	Wrists #1	106
		Thumbs #1	140
		Thumbs #2	142
		Thumbs #4	146

PROBLEM AREA	SYMPTOMS	EXERCISES	PAGE
	Lack of Strength	Wrists #1	106
		Fingers #1	128
		Fingers #4	134
		Fingers #5	135
	Tight	Forearms #3	98
		Fingers #1	128
		Fingers #3	133
		Fingers #4	134
• FINGERS •	Numb, Tingling Thumb, Index and Middle Finger	Upper Body #1	52
		Upper Body #4	60
		Upper Body #14	86
		Forearms #3	98
		Wrists #1	106
		Wrists #4	112
		Fingers #1	128
		Fingers #2	130
	Numb, Tingling Ring and Little Fingers	Upper Body #1	52
		Upper Body #9	74
		Forearms #2	96
		Wrists #1	106
		Wrists #6	118
		Wrists #9	122
		Fingers #1	128
		Thumbs #5	148

NOTES

PROFESSIONS	• Computer Operators • Data Entry Personnel • Order Entry Personnel • Telephone Operators • Travel Agents	• Accountants • Court Stenographers • Pianists • Violinists • Postal Routing Employees
MOVEMENT PATTERNS	• Rapid, repetitive movements of fingers and thumb • Wrist cocked toward little finger • Bent elbows • Stationary position for long periods of time	

	EXERCISE	PAGE
SUGGESTED EXERCISES	Upper Body #15	88
	Forearms #3	98
	Forearms #4	101
	Wrists #4	112
	Wrists #5	116
	Fingers #1	128
	Fingers #2	130
	Fingers #5	135

PREVENTION BY PROFESSION

PROFESSIONS	• Meat Processors • Poultry Processors • Carpet Layers • Glass Cutters	• Metal Workers • Welders • Mill Workers • Industrial Sewing Machine Operators
MOVEMENT PATTERNS	• Grasping • Guiding • Cutting • Arms in front of the body • Arms elevated	

SUGGESTED EXERCISES	EXERCISE	PAGE
	Upper Body #15	88
	Forearms #3	98
	Wrists #1	106
	Wrists #9	122
	Fingers #1	128
	Fingers #3	133
	Thumbs #1	140

PROFESSIONS	• Carpenters • Painters • Truck and Bus Drivers • Taxi Drivers • Homemakers • Domestic Workers	• Guitarists • Roofers • Brick Layers • Electricians • Telephone Lineworkers • Paper Hangers
MOVEMENT PATTERNS	• Grasping with the whole hand • Grasping with the fingers and thumb • Wrist flexion • Bent elbow	

	EXERCISE	PAGE
SUGGESTED EXERCISES	Upper Body #7	70
	Upper Body #11	80
	Forearms #3	98
	Forearms #5	102
	Wrists #7	120
	Fingers #1	128
	Fingers #5	135
	Thumbs #2	142
	Thumbs #6	150

PREVENTION BY PROFESSION

PROFESSIONS	• Trash Haulers • Vending Machine Operators • Shipping Clerks • Warehouse Workers • Stone Masons • Furniture Movers	
MOVEMENT PATTERNS	• Heavy lifting • Repetitive lifting • Activities requiring good grip strength	
SUGGESTED EXERCISES	EXERCISE	PAGE
	Upper Body #5	62
	Upper Body #7	70
	Upper Body #12	82
	Upper Body #13	84
	Forearms #3	98
	Forearms #5	102
	Wrists #5	116
	Wrists #7	120
	Fingers #1	128
	Fingers #3	133
	Fingers #5	135
	Thumbs #4	146

PROFESSIONS	• Beauticians • Window Washers • Teachers • Artists • Sculptors • Sign Language Interpreters	
MOVEMENT PATTERNS	• Finger and thumb action • Arms raised • Light gripping or squeezing	
SUGGESTED EXERCISES	EXERCISE	PAGE
	Upper Body #1	52
	Upper Body #5	62
	Upper Body #7	70
	Upper Body #13	84
	Upper Body #15	88
	Upper Body #16	90
	Forearms #5	102
	Fingers #1	128
	Fingers #2	130
	Fingers #5	135
	Thumbs #4	146

PROFESSIONS	• Massage Therapists • Physical Therapists • Bakers • Potters • Waiters and Waitresses
MOVEMENT PATTERNS	• Open palm pressure • Thumb activity • Lifting • Kneading

SUGGESTED EXERCISES	EXERCISE	PAGE
	Upper Body #1	52
	Upper Body #11	80
	Forearms #2	96
	Forearms #4	101
	Wrists #1	106
	Wrists #4	112
	Wrists #7	120
	Wrists #10	124
	Fingers #3	133
	Fingers #6	137
	Thumbs #4	146

PROFESSIONS	• Assemblers • Surgeons • Jewelers • Chemists • Seamstresses/Tailors • Hobbyists • Needleworkers	• Pastry Chefs • Dental Hygienists • Writers • Architects • Engineers • Microscope Technicians • Dentists
MOVEMENT PATTERNS	• Fine, precise finger and thumb movements • Elbows bent • Looking downward • Forward head	

SUGGESTED EXERCISES	EXERCISE	PAGE
	Upper Body #1	52
	Upper Body #3	58
	Upper Body #7	70
	Upper Body #11	80
	Upper Body #15	88
	Forearms #3	98
	Forearms #5	102
	Wrists #1	106
	Wrists #5	116
	Fingers #1	128
	Fingers #2	130
	Fingers #5	135

PROFESSIONS	• Power Tool Operators • Mechanics • Auto Manufacturing • Cutters • Hospital Orderlies	• Flight Attendants • Nurses • Plumbers • Maintenance Workers • Heavy Equipment Operators
MOVEMENT PATTERNS	• Gripping heavy objects while pushing • Thumb or finger action to control tools	

SUGGESTED EXERCISES	EXERCISE	PAGE
	Upper Body #7	70
	Upper Body #9	74
	Upper Body #15	88
	Forearms #2	96
	Forearms #3	98
	Wrists #1	106
	Wrists #4	112
	Wrists #6	118
	Fingers #1	128
	Fingers #3	133

PROFESSIONS	• Grocery Store Clerks • Assembly Line Packers • Catalog Order Fulfillers • Librarians
MOVEMENT PATTERNS	• Pushing with flexed wrist • Light lifting • Grasping objects less than 5 lbs.

	EXERCISE	PAGE
SUGGESTED EXERCISES	Upper Body #1	52
	Upper Body #3	58
	Upper Body #4	60
	Upper Body #11	80
	Upper Body #13	84
	Forearms #3	98
	Forearms #5	102
	Wrists #1	106
	Wrists #4	112
	Fingers #1	128
	Fingers #3	133
	Fingers #4	134
	Thumbs #1	140

PREVENTION BY PROFESSION

PROFESSIONS	• Postal Workers • File Clerks • Bank Tellers • Casino Card Dealers • Printing Press Operators • Sheet Metal Press Operators	
MOVEMENT PATTERNS	• Grasping objects between thumb and fingers • Sorting • Reaching forward	
SUGGESTED EXERCISES	EXERCISE	PAGE
	Upper Body #7	70
	Upper Body #9	74
	Upper Body #15	88
	Forearms #2	96
	Forearms #3	98
	Wrists #4	112
	Wrists #5	116
	Fingers #1	128
	Fingers #2	130
	Fingers #5	135
	Fingers #6	137
	Thumbs #4	146

PROFESSIONS	• Mothers with infant children • Students • Salespersons • Clipboard Users • Postal Delivery Personnel • Plant Supervisors	
MOVEMENT PATTERNS	• Carrying items on one arm • Bent elbow	
SUGGESTED EXERCISES	EXERCISE	PAGE
	Upper Body #1	52
	Upper Body #4	60
	Upper Body #5	62
	Upper Body #7	70
	Upper Body #9	74
	Upper Body #10	76
	Upper Body #15	88
	Forearms #3	98
	Forearms #5	102
	Wrists #5	116
	Wrists #7	120
	Fingers #3	133

NOTES

PROBLEM?	TRY THIS!
When I practice an exercise, I can't feel the Stretch Point.	When you are in position to begin the exercise, make sure your shoulders, neck, arms, and hands are relaxed. Close your eyes to help you feel sensations more completely. If you are still experiencing problems feeling the Stretch Point, refer to pages 13-16 for more information.
When I practice an exercise, I feel pain.	You are stretching too hard! Please read the section describing the Stretch Point, beginning on page 13. If the first step of an exercise causes you discomfort, discontinue using that stretch for the time being and substitute another stretch that feels easier.
My hand or fingers tingle when I am practicing a stretch.	Tingling often indicates that you are stretching muscles and connective tissue that are interfering with nerve function in that area. Any tingling you feel should be very mild and the sensation of tingling should be going away as you continue the stretch. Wiggle your fingers, wrists, and arms when you have completed the stretch.
After I practice the stretches, my muscles feel weak, tired, or sore.	You are probably stretching too hard and too often. Review the section on the Stretch Point, beginning on page 13, to make sure your technique is correct. Close your eyes as you practice the stretches to help feel the Stretch Point. Experiment with reducing the number of stretches you do in one session, and decreasing the number of times you practice the stretches each day. Try to find a balance that feels comfortable to your body. Stressing overworked tissues will delay your results.
When I am stretching, my hands go numb.	You are stretching too hard! Try finding a lighter Stretch Point so that all you feel is very light tingling. If the tingling fails to go away within ten to fifteen seconds, find another stretch which doesn't stress your body so much.

TROUBLESHOOTING

PROBLEM?	TRY THIS!
My intuition is telling me that I shouldn't stretch today.	Trust your intuition! Never stretch if it feels inappropriate. Allow yourself a break of twelve to twenty-four hours. Resume stretching when it feels "right" to you.
The exercises suggested for me don't work for my symptoms.	You may have several layers or areas of tissue that have become restricted and are causing your symptoms. Try other exercises in this book, looking for those that create a stretch in the vicinity of your problem area. You may have to release all these associated areas before the tissues that are causing your real problems can be accessed.
After I complete some of my stretches, I feel odd sensations in the areas I stretched.	Restricted connective tissues can often continue releasing after a stretch is completed. This continued releasing can feel like mild pulling, peeling, or drawing sensations. This is normal and the sensations will pass when the release is complete.
My finger, wrist, or elbow joints sometimes feel "creaky".	"Creaky" sensations can be caused by restricted tissues that function as if they were "dry". Practice the exercises suggested for your symptoms, working softly and slowly. The "creaky" sensations will gradually be replaced by a more fluid feeling as the tight tissue releases.
I am doing a stretch from the wrist section but I feel the stretch in my forearm.	Anytime a stretch is performed, it can involve tissue from other areas of the body. In this case, there probably is tissue in the forearm that must be released before the stretch can be felt in the wrist. Continue as instructed.
While I am doing some standing stretches, I feel discomfort in my back or shoulders.	Practice standing exercises in front of a mirror. Check your reflection to see if you are maintaining good posture. Often, tucking your tailbone under or dropping your shoulders is enough to correct the problem. You may also want to refer to the diagram which explains good standing posture, found on page 56.

PROBLEM?	TRY THIS!
One of my wrists can bend more than the other wrist.	Try practicing several exercises which ask you to bend your wrists separately. Examples include Wrist Exercise 7 and Wrist Exercise 8. Practice these exercises until the range of motion of your wrists is more closely matched.
I hear or feel "cracking" in my joints as I stretch.	"Cracking" joints often indicate that there are tight bands of tissue slipping across bony points as the joint moves. The "cracking" occurs when that tissue is too tight, causing it to "snap" over the bony point. This generally does not cause lasting problems but does indicate that muscle or tendon tissue in the area is too tight. Slow and gentle stretching in these areas should reduce the amount of "cracking" that is heard or felt.
When I raise my arm overhead I feel pain in the outside of my shoulder.	This type of discomfort is almost always caused by muscles in the armpit that are too tight. When the arm is raised overhead, it is necessary for muscles that pass through the armpit to lengthen, while the muscle on the outside of the shoulder (the deltoid) actually does the lifting. When the armpit area is too tight, the deltoid is asked to not only to lift the arm, but also to stretch out the restricted tissue in the armpit. This leads to fatigue in the deltoid and, ultimately, pain. Practice exercises that gently release the armpit area to reduce this type of discomfort.
I'm stretching lightly but my muscles still won't let go.	Taking slow, deep breaths can often help muscles release during a stretch. Begin the stretch by putting your body into the correct position. Inhale and imagine that your breath is completely filling the area you would like to release. Hold your breath for a count of ten and then exhale completely, pressing all air out of your lungs and squeezing your ribcage down. Repeat if necessary.
I can't stretch as far today as I could yesterday.	Muscles will change from day to day depending on how you use them. Find the Stretch Point that is appropriate for you each day.

TROUBLESHOOTING

PROBLEM?	TRY THIS!
My hands go numb while I am asleep.	Many people curl their hands under at the wrist as they sleep. This can aggravate muscles that have become short and tight on the inside of the forearm. Nerves passing through the area at the front of the shoulder can also become pinched by this sleeping position. Before going to bed, practice the exercises for the inside of the forearm and the armpit (see the "Which Exercises Should I Do?" section). Many people will also find it helpful to hug a thick pillow while they sleep. This prevents the hands from curling under and the shoulders from rolling forward toward the center of the chest.
I no longer feel symptoms while I am at work but symptoms soon return when I resume my favorite hobbies.	Hobbies and work activities can affect the muscles and connective tissues differently. It is important to focus on each symptom separately so the tissues creating the symptom can be individually helped. Find the appropriate exercises for symptoms created by your hobbies (see the "Which Exercises Should I Do?" section) and practice those exercises as well as the exercises you are doing for your work-related symptoms.
My symptoms recur when I stop doing the exercises consistently.	It is important to continually prepare your muscles and connective tissues for the strains they are being asked to withstand. Practicing the exercises recommended for your symptoms is the best way to condition your body for daily activities. Read "How Often Should I Stretch?" found on pages 18 for further information.
I stretch consistently but my symptoms come back quickly.	Muscle and connective tissue runs in many layers through the body. If your symptoms return quickly, this often indicates that there are deeper layers of tissue that have not been completely released. Every time you practice your stretches, hold each position longer, allowing several stretch points to develop and then release before going on to the next stretch.

THE EXERCISES

The exercises in this program are divided into five groups according to the area of the body they are designed to help: Upper Body, Forearms, Wrists, Fingers, and Thumbs. Try each of the exercises to find the ones that help relieve the symptoms you experience. For further guidance in choosing appropriate exercises, please consult the "Charts" section beginning on page 23.

NOTES

. . . .

UPPER BODY

Most people spend very little time thinking about the upper body - that is, until our neck, shoulders, chest, upper back, or sides begin to develop painful symptoms.

At least 50 percent of all people suffering from Carpal Tunnel Syndrome or repetitive strain injuries are living with afflicted muscles and connective tissues of the upper body. When these tissues are restored to their normal loose and fluid state, there is a significant reduction in the symptoms that remain.

The exercises in this section are designed to help restore the soft tissues of the upper body to a more natural state. Best results will be achieved if you incorporate several of them into your daily routine.

UPPER BODY

· ·

EXERCISE 1

- *Restores mobility to neck*
- *Lengthens short and tight neck and shoulder muscles*
- *Reduces the opportunity for nerve compression at the neck*

Treat painful tissue with the utmost care and kindness. Practice this exercise slowly and thoughtfully.

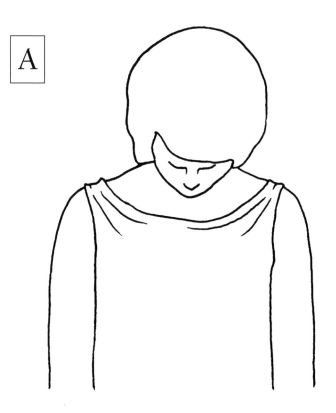

A

- Stand or sit comfortably with your shoulders relaxed.
- Drop your head forward and wait there, noticing the stretch point that appears at the back of your neck.
- Wait in this position until the stretch point releases.

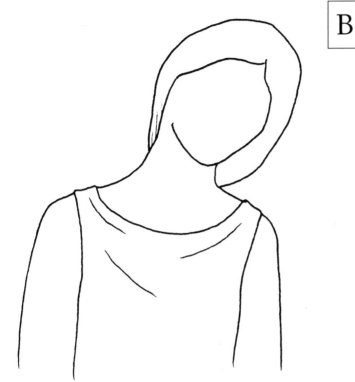

B

Hint: Try propping your head in your hand as you do this exercise. This will limit the pull on overly tight neck muscles and will make the release easier to accomplish.

• Roll your head one inch to the left. Notice the new muscle fibers being stretched in this position.

• Hold this position until you feel the stretch point release.

• Roll your head another one inch to the left and wait for the release.

Exercise 1

Free movement of the shoulder joint and the neck are important to people who participate in sports such as golf, tennis, baseball, squash, and swimming. Practicing the exercises offered in this section of the program will help promote optimum function of the upper body as well as prolong the number of years an athlete can actively participate in these sports.

C

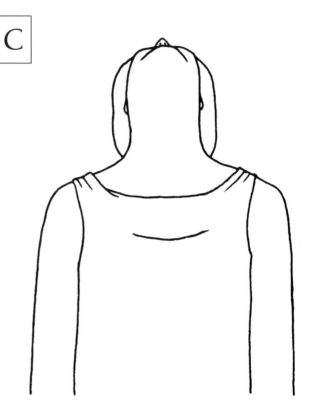

- Slowly work your way around to complete one full circle.
- Keep the shoulders level and relaxed.

BODY AWARENESS

Stand Up Straight!

One of the most common ways we misuse our bodies is in our standing posture. When was the last time you felt uplifted, energetic, and at the same time, solidly grounded while standing?

Here are some simple techniques that can help you regain a more natural balance when you stand. Practice them when you are standing still as well as when you are walking. You will soon gain a new sense of energy, vitality, and balance.

1. Stand with your usual posture. Have a friend stand behind you and press down firmly on your shoulders simulating the effect of gravity. Does your body collapse in the middle under the pressure? If it does, then you are not stacking the sections of your body squarely on top of one another. With each step you take, gravity has the opportunity to pull you down, creating stresses on muscles and joints.

2. Stand once again with your usual posture. Look down at your feet. Adjust your position until you can see where your feet and ankles meet. Keeping your body in the same position from the torso down, lift only your head to look straight ahead. Have your friend press down on your shoulders once again. Does your body feel more solidly aligned?

An aligned standing posture is the foundation for effecting change in Carpal Tunnel Syndrome and other repetitive strain injuries. When you stand up straight, all of your bones and muscles fall into their natural alignment. This allows plenty of room for the nerves (which can create the symptoms of Carpal Tunnel Syndrome or other repetitive strain injuries) to pass through the body unimpeded.

There are many holding patterns that can ultimately cause bad posture. Here are a few:

• Forward head

• Shoulders rolled forward

• Shoulders pulled back

• Depressed chest

• Puffed-out chest

• Overly tight stomach muscles

• Tight, arched low back

• Rigid, inflexible spine

• Elbows pulled back

• Knees pointing outward

• Knees pointing inward

• Feet pointing outward

Each of these postural deviations are created by habit, injury, or other trauma to the soft tissues, the muscles, and connective tissues of the body. The problems they create are compounded by our lack of awareness about how to hold our bodies.

BODY AWARENESS

Look In The Mirror!

The diagrams below illustrate two possible standing postures. Which posture appears more supportive?

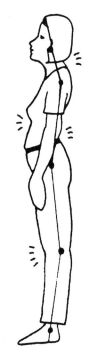

The person with this posture is experiencing a great deal of discomfort: Her forward head is creating a significant amount of neck pain, the depressed position of her ribcage is limiting the amount of breath she can take in, the extra curvature of her lower back is pinching her spinal discs and leading to back pain and injury.

This person is having an entirely different experience. Each section of her body is sitting squarely upon the one below, creating support and stability. Her hips are relaxed with no lower back compression. Her chest is open, allowing for full breaths which will bring plenty of oxygen to her brain and muscles. Her head is sitting properly on her shoulders. In this position, she will be less likely to experience neck and shoulder pain.

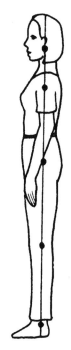

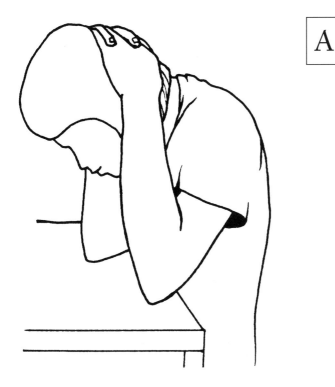

A

* *Lengthens muscles at the back of the neck*
* *Stretches the trapezius muscle in the upper back*

* Interlace your fingers and place them at the back of your head.
* Tilt your head forward, bringing your chin to your chest.
* Do not pull forward with your hands. Rather, allow the weight of your arms to help create the stretch.
* The exercise is complete when you feel a "softening" at the back of the neck.

UPPER BODY

. . . .

EXERCISE 3

- Reduces general shoulder

  tension

- Helps create awareness of

  unconscious holding in

  the shoulders

Hint: If you allow your arms to hang loosely as you do this exercise you should experience a good stretch through the upper arms as well as through the upper shoulders.

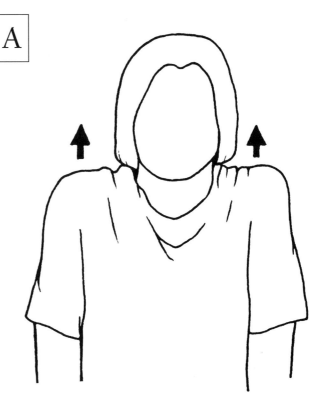

A

- Allow your arms to hang relaxed by your sides.
- Shrug your shoulders upward, trying to touch your ears with the tops of your shoulders.
- Hold this position for five to ten seconds.

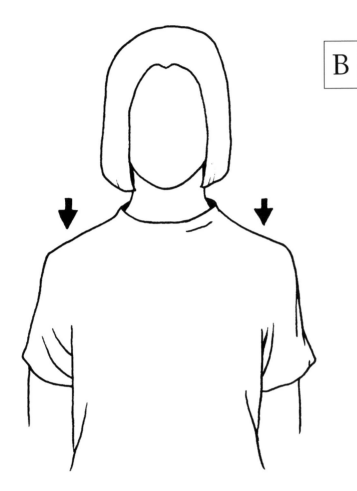

B

- Slowly pull your shoulders down, away from your ears, as far as they will go.
- Hold this position for five to ten seconds.

EXERCISE 3

The median nerve, which is responsible for much of the misery in repetitive strain injuries, especially Carpal Tunnel Syndrome, leaves the spine from a point in the neck. It is possible for the nerve to be compressed at many points along its route through the shoulder, down the arm, through the carpal tunnel, and into the hand. Exercises to relieve tension in the muscles of the upper body are highly recommended as part of a daily exercise routine to ensure that the nerve passes through these areas without interference.

EXERCISE 4

- *Lengthens muscles at the side of the neck*

- *Stretches upper shoulder and upper arm*

To get the best results possible with this exercise program, pay careful attention to the Stretch Point and Release. See pages 13-18 for complete information.

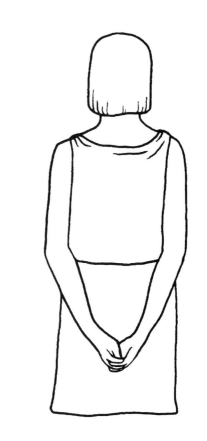

A

- Clasp your hands behind your back at hip level.

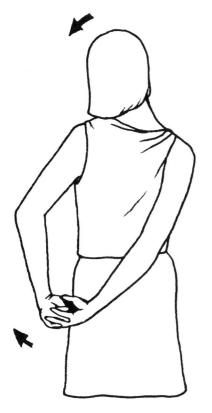

B

Hint: You can create further exercise variations by rolling your head one inch to the front or back while it is tilted to the side.

- With your shoulders down and relaxed, pull your clasped hands to the left.

- Tilt your head to the left, bringing your left ear and your left shoulder closer.

- Notice the stretch point that appears at the side of your neck.

- Wait for the release.

- Repeat this exercise to the right.

UPPER BODY

EXERCISE 5

- Relieves tension between

    the shoulder blades

- Mobilizes shoulder blades

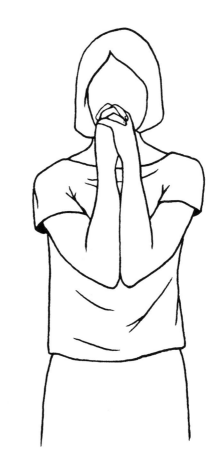

A

- Clasp your hands together, interlocking your

    fingers.

- Bring your elbows together, imagining they are

    glued to each other.

- This position will often bring on a stretch point.

- Wait for the release before proceeding.

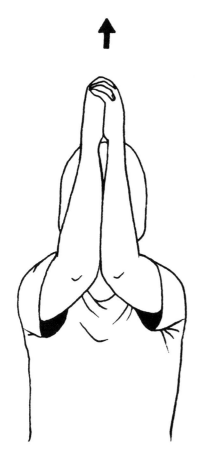

B

Hint: This exercise is easier while on your back in bed. What a great way to begin or end your day!

- With your elbows pressed together, lift your

  forearms toward the ceiling.

- Pause at the first sign of a stretch point.

- Wait for the release.

EXERCISE 5

Pain and restriction between the shoulder blades is a common complaint of people who work at a desk. Widening the space between the shoulder blades and then moving them through their range of motion can be a very effective way to release tension in this area. This is a great exercise to get the job done.

C

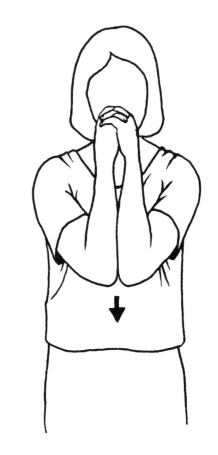

- Return your arms to the beginning position of the exercise.

- Keeping your elbows together, pull your forearms down.

- Hold this position until the stretch point releases.

BODY AWARENESS

Sitting Your Way To Comfort

Most of us spend very little time paying attention to how we sit, and how we feel when we sit. Here are a few suggestions to increase your awareness of how you feel in a chair, sofa, or car:

1. Sit in your usual way, in the seat of your choice. Consider your body in terms of alignment. Does your body feel straight or do you feel twisted? Are both hips squarely on the seat? Are your shoulders level? Is your neck comfortable? Do you have a sense of support in your body?

2. Still sitting in your usual way, take a deep breath. Notice the volume of breath you can take in. Notice how your body feels as you inhale. Does this position create the possibility of taking deep, full breaths? Now, sit in a straight position. Again, take a deep breath. Is it any easier than before? Were you able to take in more air? Does this posture make it easier to breathe fully?

3. Sit in a slouched position. Turn your head to the left and the right. Notice how far you can go in each direction. Notice how your neck feels as you turn. Now, sit in a more upright position. Again, turn your head in both directions. Feel the difference? Which option would create less neck pain?

Sitting in a slouched or unbalanced position can contribute to stress in the workplace. Slouching or twisting through the torso can cause compression of the ribcage which, in turn, can interfere with the ability to breathe fully and easily. If we consistently take shallow breaths we rob the brain of the oxygen it requires for quick thinking and rapid response. Lack of oxygen can also lead to muscle fatigue since oxygen is an important component in muscle metabolism. Do you ever wonder why you feel bone-tired after a day of sitting and working at a desk?

A simple way of reducing stress on the job is to sit properly and take full, complete breaths throughout your day. You will have more energy to handle the rigors of today's working world.

EXERCISE 6

- *Reduces tension in the upper back*
- *Helps stretch deep muscles at the side of the neck*

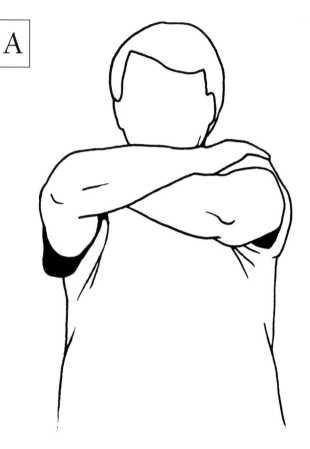

A

- Place your hands on opposite shoulders.
- Point your elbows straight out in front of your body.

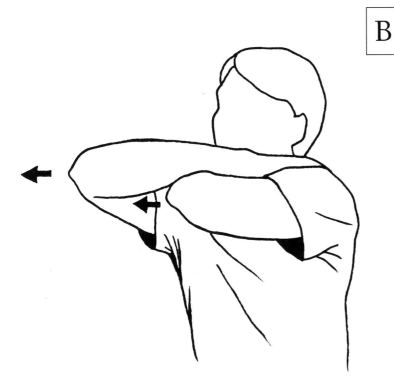

B

Exercise 6

Until Carpal Tunnel Syndrome and repetitive strain injuries became prominent in the mid-1980s, one of the biggest occupational complaints was chronic neck and shoulder pain. These problems still exist. The exercises in this section can be very helpful for relieving this type of pain.

- Pull your elbows straight out and away from your body.

- Notice the stretch point and wait for the release.

UPPER BODY

EXERCISE 6

Tight muscles and tendons respond best to slow, comfortable stretching.

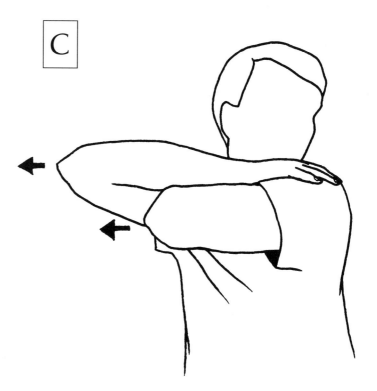

- While your elbows are extended forward, try turning your head to the left.
- Notice the stretch point that appears and wait for the release.
- Repeat by turning your head to the right.

BODY AWARENESS

Getting To Know Your Shoulders

The shoulders are an area of the body we seldom pay attention to...until they become painful. Those who sit for most of the day will be all too familiar with discomfort in their shoulders. Here are a few awareness exercises to help familiarize you with this important area of your body:

1. Pull one shoulder forward and one shoulder back. Try to keep your torso pointing straight ahead. Now reverse this pattern and notice if one combination is easier than the other.

2. Shrug one shoulder up toward your ear. Did the other shoulder try to raise at the same time? With one shoulder up, pull the other shoulder down. With one smooth movement, try to switch this pattern. Can you do it?

3. Move one shoulder in a backward circle. Does your other shoulder tense up or want to help with this movement? Repeat this exercise with the other shoulder. What do you notice now? Here's a hard one - try rotating one shoulder in a backward direction, the other in a forward direction. What do you notice?

4. Inhale, allowing your ribcage to expand and your shoulders to rise up toward your ears. Now exhale, fully deflating your ribs but keeping your shoulders up. Tricky, isn't it?

The shoulder girdle is made up of only four bones - two collarbones and two shoulder blades. These bones are "floating" in muscle at the front, sides, and back of the body. The bones are attached to the torso by means of two small cartilage joints at the "notch" between the collarbones. Ideally, the shoulder girdle should have free and separate movement in relation to the ribcage and spine.

As we age, many of us develop movement patterns that link together the movement of the shoulder girdle and the torso. This can lead to increased tension, fatigue, and limited range of motion. This restriction continues to build as the habitual holding pattern persists and the fascia in the area becomes increasingly tight and sticky.

It is important to continually try to break up habitual movement patterns to avoid this gradual loss of function. Try the body awareness exercises suggested here and throughout the book to learn more about your body and how you use it. You can also learn about yourself by creating your own ways to mix up your movement patterns. It's fun to discover new ways to accomplish old tasks.

Your body will thank you.

UPPER BODY

EXERCISE 7

- Reduces general shoulder tension

- Keeps shoulders loose and flexible

- Increases awareness of tension build-up in the shoulder

Success with this program is greatly enhanced the more you understand how your body becomes injured and how healing changes can be made to damaged tissue. Please read the section titled "Self-Care Success" beginning on page 1 to maximize your results.

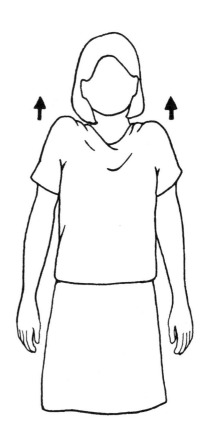

A

- Raise your shoulders up toward your ears.
- Allow your arms to hang loosely at your sides.

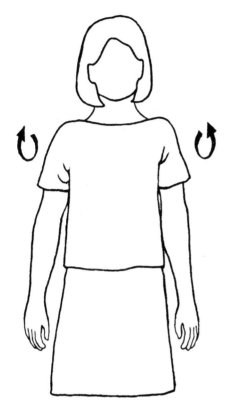

B

EXERCISE 7

As we go through life, most of us create movement patterns that become automatic and limited in range of motion. We move our joints in ways that we have become used to. This exercise can help you recognize new directions to move your shoulders. See if you can create other movement combinations for your shoulders that feel new and different.

- Very slowly rotate your shoulders toward the front of your body.

- Continue rotating your shoulders down to the lowest point.

- Continue around to the back and return to the starting position.

- Make the widest circle possible.

- Perform another complete revolution in the opposite direction.

EXERCISE 8

- Excellent stretch for the underarm area

- Stretches many of the rotator cuff muscles

- Lengthens the triceps in the upper arm

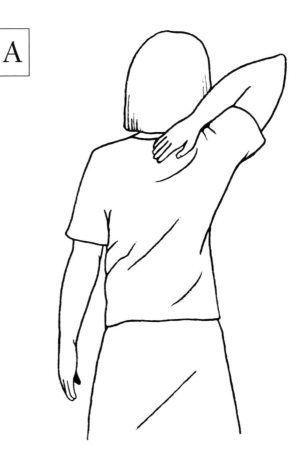

A

- Place your hand at the base of your neck, palm flat.

- Extend your elbow out to the side, in a straight line with your shoulder and ear.

- Hold this position for ten seconds.

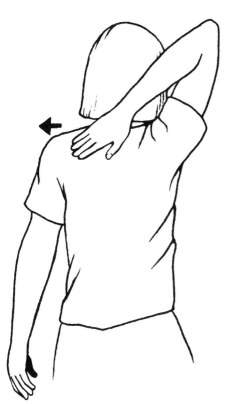

B

EXERCISE 8

- Slowly slide your hand toward the opposite shoulder.

- Try to keep your shoulder down and relaxed.

- Pause at the stretch point and wait for the release.

The armpit is an area that we seldom pay attention to but can be the site of major muscular holding problems. Tight muscles passing through the armpit can interfere with your ability to raise your arm to brush your teeth or comb your hair. They can also make it almost impossible to relax your shoulders and can even affect your ability to take a full, deep breath. Releasing this area is important for conquering Carpal Tunnel Syndrome and other repetitive strain injuries of the upper body.

UPPER BODY

. . . .

EXERCISE 9

- Lengthens muscles at the side of the torso

- Great stretch for the "lats" (the latissimus dorsi muscle)

- Stretches the upper arms

Hint: You can achieve a more thorough stretch by propping your lower elbow on a table, pillow, or other surface as you bend to the side. This allows the weight of your upper body to be fully supported, creating the opportunity to let go of all other muscles as you stretch.

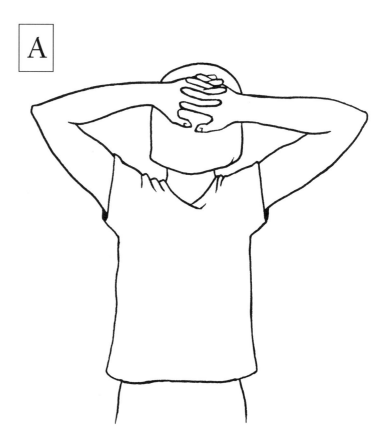

A

- Lace your fingers together and place them behind your head.

- Hold your elbows wide out to the side, in line with your ears and shoulders.

- Do not go on to the next step until you can do this step without discomfort.

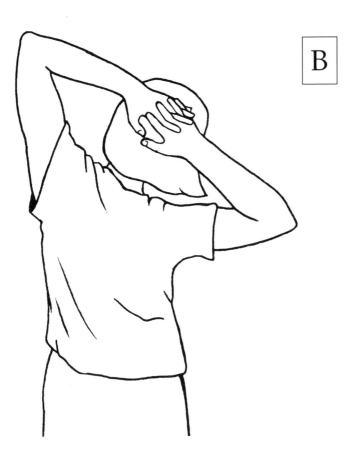

B

EXERCISE 9

Hint: For an advanced stretch, try moving your elbow three inches forward as you pull it up toward the ceiling. This creates a good stretch in the armpit area.

- Tilt your body to the right, pulling your left elbow up toward the ceiling.

- Keep your neck as relaxed as possible.

- Return to the starting position and repeat to the other side.

UPPER BODY

EXERCISE 10

- Helps maintain mobility of the shoulder joints

- Stretches the back of the arms

- Moves upper back muscles through a wide range of motion

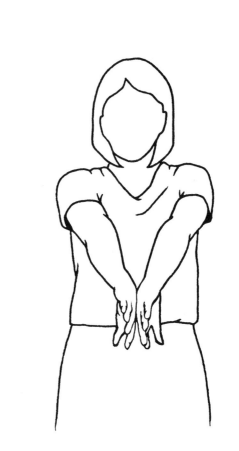

A

- Extend your arms straight in front of your body with your elbows comfortably straight but not locked.

- Turn your arms so the backs of your hands touch, palms out.

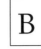

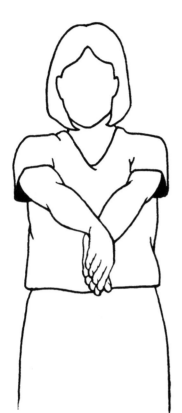

Hint: This stretch is easy to do while on your back in bed.

- Criss-cross your arms so the palms are pressed against one another.

- Hold this position for several seconds.

UPPER BODY

EXERCISE 10

Hint: While lying on your back in bed you can create a variation of this stretch. Try stretching one leg downward through the heel while your arms are stretched overhead. Repeat with the other leg.

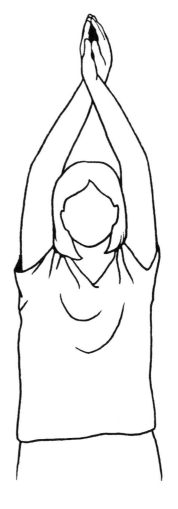

- Raise your arms straight over your head, fingertips pointing toward the ceiling.
- Keep your shoulders down and relaxed.
- Repeat this exercise by crossing your hands in the opposite direction.

BODY AWARENESS

Our Habitual Movement Patterns

As human beings we are creatures of habit. As we age, it becomes increasingly difficult to distinguish between movements that have become our habits and movements that are part of our body's natural design. The constant repetition of habitual movement patterns causes changes in the soft tissues of the body, primarily the fascia. Over time, these tissues become short and tight, reflecting our movement habits. In recovering from any repetitive strain injury, it is important that we discover as many of our movement habits as possible and change them. Moving in new ways helps free tight and restricted tissues and keeps our bodies in a loose and fluid condition. Try the following examples of common movement habits:

1. Fold your arms across your chest in the way most usual for you. Notice that your body feels comfortable in this position. Now reverse the way your arms are crossed. Many people will find it difficult to figure out how to create this reversal. Notice how unusual it feels to have your arms crossed in this new way.

2. Sit with your legs crossed and notice how "at home" your body feels in this position. Now switch, crossing your legs in the opposite way. Allow your body to completely relax in this new position. Notice the changes your body goes through trying to get used to the new pattern.

Habitual movement and holding patterns are evident in all areas of our lives. For example, cradling the phone on a shoulder or shrugging to rest on the armrest of a chair that is too high causes tension in the body. Other common patterns include adopting a stiff posture when we don a suit for work, tightening up our stomachs and knees when wearing high-heeled shoes, shrugging one shoulder to carry a briefcase or shoulder bag. We incorporate these patterns so thoroughly they become second nature to us.

To more easily discover the patterns you have adopted, begin to think of your body in terms of balance. Notice if you continually lean to one side, lift or carry objects using the same hand, or balance more weight on one foot than the other. As you pay attention to the patterns you have adopted, you will find they are actually uncomfortable. You will be reminded to change whenever you feel this discomfort.

EXERCISE 11

- *Stretches entire inside of arm*

- *Increases wrist flexibility*

- *Lengthens finger tendons*

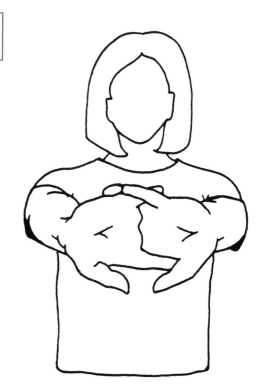

A

- Fold your hands, fingers interlaced.

- Turn your hands over and push your palms away from your body.

- This step creates a strong stretch for the palms and fingers. Be careful not to overstretch!

- Do not go on to the next step until you can do this step without discomfort.

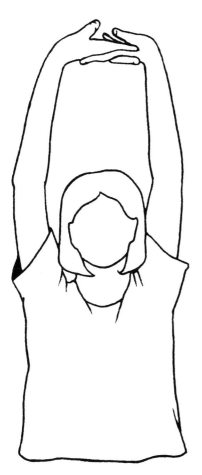

B

EXERCISE 11

Hint: You can vary this exercise by using your breath. With your arms stretched overhead, take a deep breath and hold it until you feel your muscles soften into a release. Then exhale, pushing all the breath out of your lungs. Hold this position until you feel a release.

- Slowly raise your arms until they are extended straight over your head.

- Keep your back straight, not arched.

- Try this exercise while lying on your back in bed.

EXERCISE 12

- *Great stretch for the whole spine*
- *Reduces lower back tension*

The bones of the spine, the vertebrae, are meant to move every time we move. However, over the course of our lives, most of us stiffen up and we end up moving as if we have a pole for a spinal column. This exercise helps restore flexibility to the spine by creating a gentle "wringing" motion. Try it, it feels great!

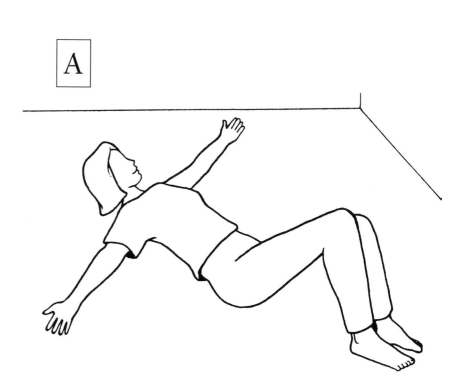

A

- Lie on the floor with your knees bent and feet together.
- Extend your arms straight out to the side, palms up.

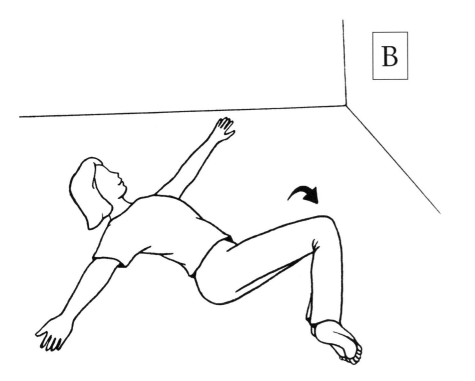

B

EXERCISE 12

Hint: If you find it difficult to roll your knees all the way over to the floor as illustrated in the exercise, place one or two pillows so your knees will land on them as they roll to the side. Fully relax into this position to get the full benefit of this gentle stretch. Then, as your muscles lengthen, you can take away the pillows and slowly work toward achieving the full stretch.

- Roll your knees to the left, toward the floor.
- Turn your left palm down. Your right palm should remain facing the ceiling.
- Take a deep breath and relax into this position.
- Return to the starting position and repeat to the other side.

UPPER BODY

EXERCISE 13

- *Stretches side of the torso*

- *Restores mobility to the ribcage*

- *Significantly reduces tension in the shoulders*

Overworked tissues repair faster when they are stretched softly and carefully. See pages 13 - 16 for more information.

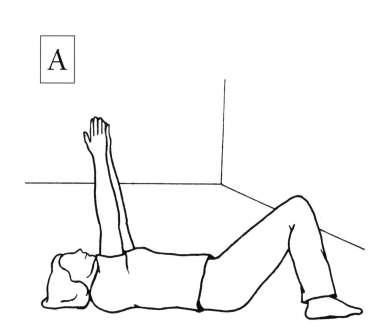

A

- Lie on the floor with your knees bent and your feet about hip-width apart.

- Place your palms together and extend your arms and fingertips toward the ceiling.

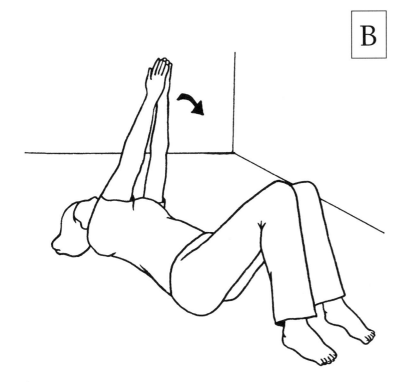

B

The latissimus, a large, flat muscle extending from the lower back to the upper arm is often involved in shoulder pain and discomfort. This is an excellent exercise for releasing the latissimus and for improving the range of motion of the ribcage and shoulders.

- With your palms firmly together, roll your arms and shoulders to the left.

- Your hips should remain on the floor.

- Take a deep breath and relax your head, neck, and spine.

- For variation, try raising your arms so your finger tips are extended slightly above the level of your forehead.

UPPER BODY

. . . .

EXERCISE 14

- Improves posture

- Lengthens muscles of the chest

- Reduces tension in the underarm area

- Stretches upper arms

Hint: If you are not tall enough to reach the doorframe above your head, consider buying and installing a chin-up bar in a doorway, at a height that is easy for you to reach.

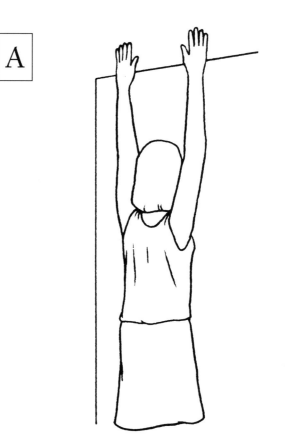

A

- Standing in a doorway, raise your arms overhead and hold the doorframe above you.

- Elbows should be straight, but not locked.

- Keep your shoulders down and relaxed.

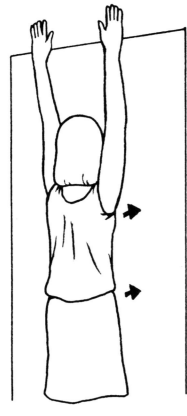

B

Many of us have developed a habit of slouching as we sit or even as we stand. Shortness in the muscles and fascia at the front of the body can greatly contribute to slouching. This exercise is great for stretching the front of the body and helping to eliminate that forward droop.

- Take a half step forward.

- Keep your hips in line directly under your shoulders.

- Take a deep breath, inflating your ribcage fully.

- For variation, turn your head to the left, take a deep breath, and hold until you feel a release.

- Repeat to the right.

UPPER BODY

EXERCISE 15

- Stretches upper chest

- Improves breathing

- Improves posture

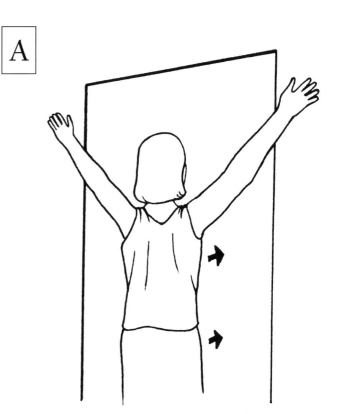

A

- Standing in a doorway, place your hands at the ten o'clock and two o'clock positions on the doorjamb.

- Take a half step forward until you feel a stretch point.

- Keep your body in a straight line with your hips directly under your shoulders.

- Take a deep breath, hold, then exhale completely to encourage the release.

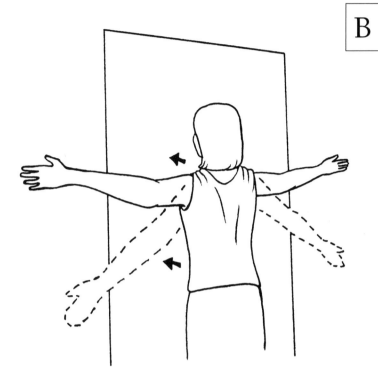

B

EXERCISE 15

- Place your hands at the three o'clock and nine o'clock positions.

- Repeat the stretching process in Step A.

- Place your hands at the five o'clock and seven o'clock positions.

- Repeat the stretch as in Step A.

The median nerve is responsible for the majority of Carpal Tunnel Syndrome symptoms. It passes directly under the pectoral muscles, the large muscles at the upper chest, on its way to the hands. Keeping the pectoral muscles loose and unrestricted can reduce the possibility of nerves being pinched at the shoulder.

UPPER BODY

EXERCISE 16

- *Stretches deep shoulder muscles*

- *Mobilizes shoulder blades*

- *Lengthens muscles at the back of the shoulders*

Closing your eyes while you practice these stretches will help you develop an awareness of the subtleties of the Stretch Point. Learn more about the Stretch Point beginning on page 13.

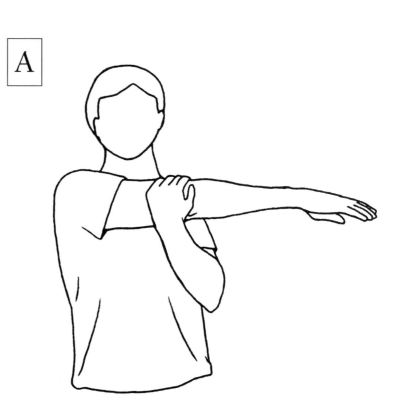

A

- Draw your arm straight across your body.
- Hold your arm just above the elbow for support.
- Gently pull your arm closer to your body.
- Hold this position until you feel a release.

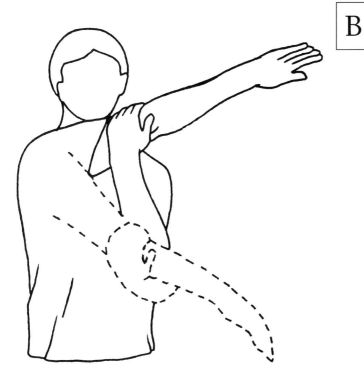

B

EXERCISE 16

Most people will find they are able to stretch the muscles on one side of their body farther or more easily than on the other side. It is also common for muscles to stretch to a certain level on one day and less on the next. This is normal and relates to the kind of stresses to which that area of your body is routinely subjected.

Always honor the limits your body has on any given day. Never overstretch just to have the same range of motion from side to side or from day to day. With gentle practice, the range of motion of your muscles will begin to even out all by themselves.

- From the starting position, lift your arm up until your hand is at forehead level.
- Pull your arm closer, hold, and wait for the release.
- From the beginning position, pull your arm down until your hand is at waist height.
- Pull your arm closer to your body, hold, and wait for the release.

FOREARMS

Almost every person suffering from Carpal Tunnel Syndrome and other repetitive strain injuries has significant changes to the muscles and connective tissues in the forearms. After all, the muscles that move the wrist and fingers are chiefly located in the forearms near the elbow. If you lay your fingers across the widest part of your forearm and wiggle the fingers of your free hand, you should feel the separate movement of the forearm muscles. If you do not feel the rippling of your muscles in this area, this may indicate that adhesions have formed in the fascia between the muscles and is generally the result of repetitive or strained activities. This condition creates fatigue and a feeling of weakness in the forearms and fingers.

The exercises in this section will help you restore free and easy movement to the muscles of your forearm. With careful practice, you may also experience a return of your original strength as the tissues relax and lengthen.

FOREARMS

EXERCISE 1

- *Stretches the outside edge of the forearm from elbow to hand*

- *Begins to loosen deep tendons of the thumb*

Carefully read the instructions for each exercise you decide to include in your routine. The instructions contain helpful guidance, necessary for achieving the best possible results.

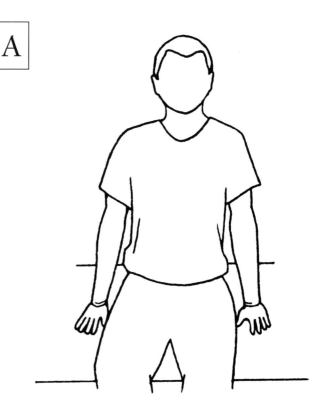

A

- While seated, place your hands on either side of your body, fingers pointing forward, palms down.
- Keep your elbows straight without locking them.
- Make sure you are sitting up straight!

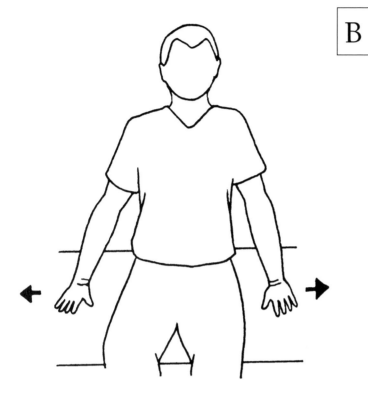

B

EXERCISE 1

Many of the tissue changes in muscle and fascia seen in Carpal Tunnel Syndrome and other repetitive strain injuries occur along the ulna bone in the forearm which helps form the elbow. This exercise, practiced gently, helps restore these tissues to a more normal state.

- Slowly slide your hands out to the side while keeping your palms flat.

- Pause when you feel the stretch point anywhere in your fingers, hands, wrists, or forearms.

- Hold this position until you feel the release.

FOREARMS

EXERCISE 2

- Lengthens finger tendons

- Restores wrist flexibility

- Helps relieve elbow pain

The more slowly and softly you practice this stretch, the faster you will achieve positive results.

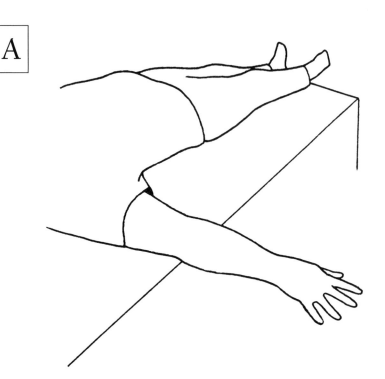

A

- Lie comfortably near the edge of a bed with your elbow well supported and several inches away from the edge.

- Your palm should be facing down and your fingers spread wide open.

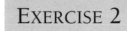

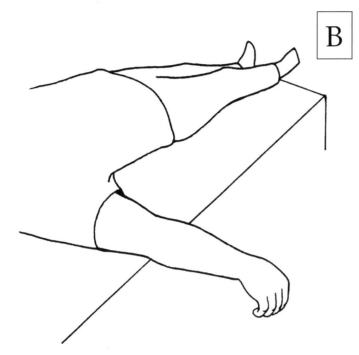

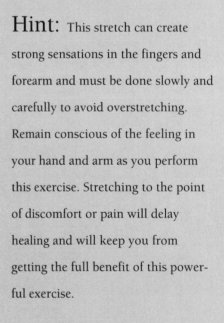

Hint: This stretch can create strong sensations in the fingers and forearm and must be done slowly and carefully to avoid overstretching. Remain conscious of the feeling in your hand and arm as you perform this exercise. Stretching to the point of discomfort or pain will delay healing and will keep you from getting the full benefit of this powerful exercise.

- Curl your fingers and hand under into a claw shape, one inch at a time.

- Pause at each stretch point and wait for the release.

- End the exercise when your fingers are closed in a fist and your wrist is fully bent.

FOREARMS

EXERCISE 3

- *Lengthens tendons and muscles on the inside of the forearm*
- *Helps relieve elbow pain*

The stretch points in this exercise will often feel like a deep ache. This is perfectly normal. If the aching sensation becomes uncomfortable, simply move your body toward the center of the bed. This will allow your elbow to be supported more by the bed and should create a more comfortable sensation.

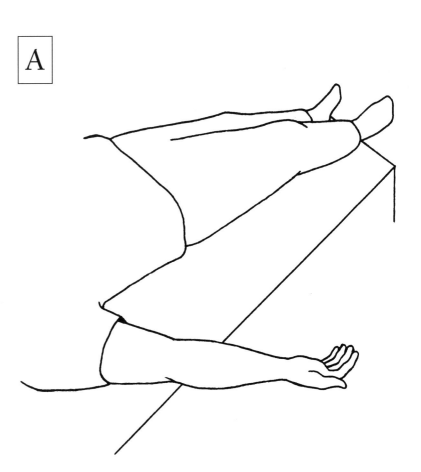

A

- Lie face up on a bed with your arm straight out to the side, palm up.
- Hang your arm off the side of the bed making sure your elbow is well supported and several inches from the edge.
- Relax all of your muscles, especially your fingers.
- If this position creates a stretch point, allow it to release and lengthen before continuing.

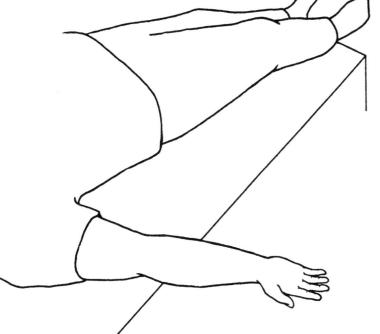
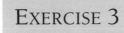

EXERCISE 3

Those who suffer from Carpal Tunnel Syndrome not only experience nerve pain at the wrist, but also pain and restriction in the muscles of the forearm. Even though this exercise can take longer than most to complete, it is one of the very best for relieving pain in the forearms. Try it at least once to see if it does the trick for you.

- Open your fingers about one inch. Wait in this position for a new stretch point to develop and then disappear.

- Continue opening your fingers in one inch increments until your hand is fully open.

- Give your body plenty of time to get the full benefit of this stretch.

FOREARMS

EXERCISE 3

This is an advanced form of the same stretch. Please be sure that you can comfortably perform the previous two steps before attempting this stretch.

Some people occasionally feel tingling in their fingertips while performing this stretch. This generally indicates that tissues interfering with the function of the nerve are being stretched. If you should feel this tingling, reduce the amount of stretch until the tingling sensation is very light.* In a short period of time (ten to fifteen seconds), the tingling should disappear. If it does not, then soften the stretch even more. Discontinue this stretch if you feel any numbness. Substitute the upper body stretches of your choice.

* See "What is the Stretch Point" on page 13.

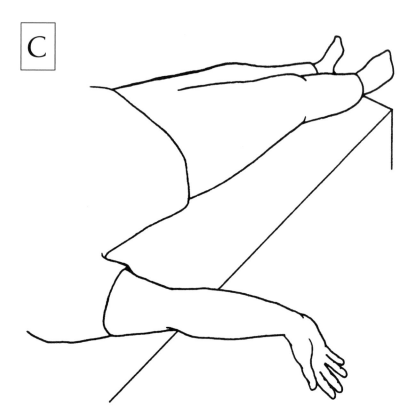

- Spread your fingers wide apart and wait for the new stretch point to release.
- Keeping your fingers straight and apart, bend your wrist back about one inch.
- Continue bending your wrist back in one inch increments, waiting for the release, until your wrist is fully extended.

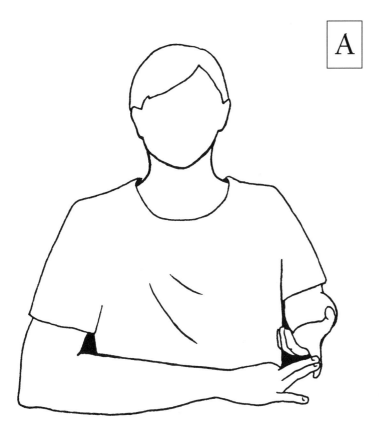

A

EXERCISE 4

- *Releases the deepest muscles of the inner forearm*
- *Reduces the fatigue created by most finger activities*
- *Restores strength and endurance to the forearm muscles*

Hint: This exercise is very important to anyone who uses extensive finger action in their work. These jobs would include keyboard operators, assemblers, surgeons, musicians, students, teachers, crafters, mechanics, construction workers, and many more. Try this exercise a few times to see if it meets your needs.

- Gently rest your forearm parallel to your body, palm down, on a table or desk.
- Do not lean any weight on your arm.
- Fingers should remain relaxed.
- With your other hand, gently lift the middle and ring fingers, just to the point where the other fingers begin to lift off the table surface.
- Hold this subtle stretch until you feel a release.

FOREARMS

EXERCISE 5

- *Helps relieve numbness in ring and little fingers*
- *Stretches the outside of the forearm to the elbow*
- *Increases wrist flexibility*

It might take several sessions before you can stretch your arms to this level position. Please be patient. It is important that you allow your muscles plenty of time to be restored to their natural flexibility.

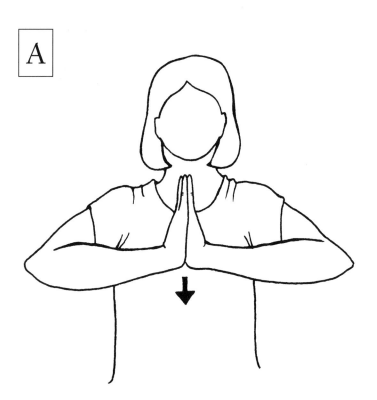

A

- With your hands together in a praying position, fingers relaxed, press the heels of your palms down and stop at the stretch point. Hold until you feel the release.
- Continue pressing the heels of your palms down in small increments until your wrists are level with your elbows.
- Do not go on to the next step until you can complete this step in total comfort.

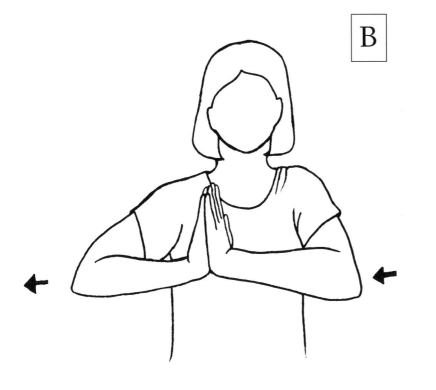

B

EXERCISE 5

Muscles and tendons that are causing you pain have been working hard for you for a long time. Gently encouraging them to stretch and lengthen will restore them to health in the quickest way possible.

- Once the heels of your palms are level with your elbows, shift your hands, arms, and elbows to the right until you feel the first stretch point.

- Pause in this position and wait for the stretch point to release.

- Return to the starting position and repeat by shifting to the left.

NOTES

・・・

WRISTS

Think of the wrist as a flexible junction. Muscles that start in the forearm become tendons just before they reach the wrist. At the wrist these tendons pass under two bracelets of connective tissue known as the retinaculae. Muscles on the top side of the forearm (in line with the back of the hand) generally cause the fingers to lift up. Muscles on the underside of the forearm (the palm side) cause the fingers to bend toward the palm.

It is essential that tendons be able to move easily under the retinaculae to prevent many of the symptoms of Carpal Tunnel Syndrome. Exercises in this section are specifically designed to facilitate this movement.

WRISTS

· · · · · · · · · · · · · · · · · ·

Exercise 1

- Helps restore freedom of

  movement to fingers

- Improves wrist flexibility

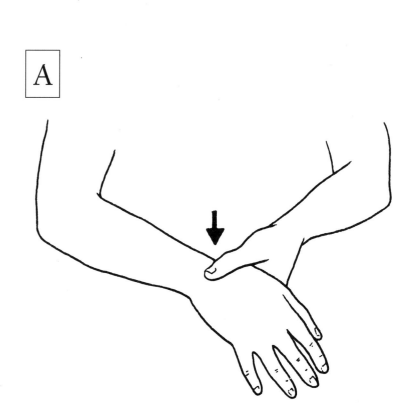

A

- Grasp your right wrist firmly with your left hand. Your thumb will be on top of your wrist and the rest of your fingers will be underneath.

- Press your thumb into the back of your wrist using the same pressure it would take to make a dent in a tennis ball.

- Reduce the pressure slightly if this causes any discomfort.

B

EXERCISE 1

This "Wrist Release" exercise helps release a bracelet of connective tissue surrounding the wrist called the Extensor Retinaculum. This bracelet of tissue becomes "sticky" when strained by repetitive motion and can prevent tissues from gliding easily under it. Releasing this area can help reduce many of the symptoms associated with Carpal Tunnel Syndrome.

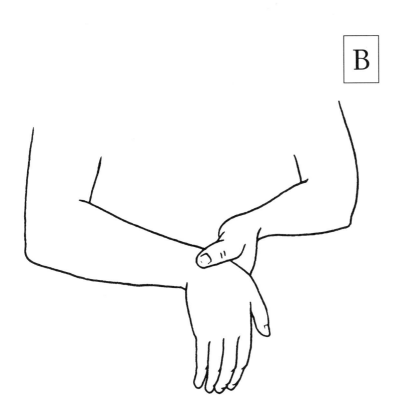

- Keeping your thumb stationary, slowly bend your wrist down, allowing the skin of your wrist to slide under your thumb.

- Repeat this pattern until you have covered the entire top surface of your wrist.

WRISTS

· · · · · · · · · · · · · · · · · · ·

Exercise 2

- Increases range of motion of the wrist
- Stretches all muscles and tendons which cross the wrist

A

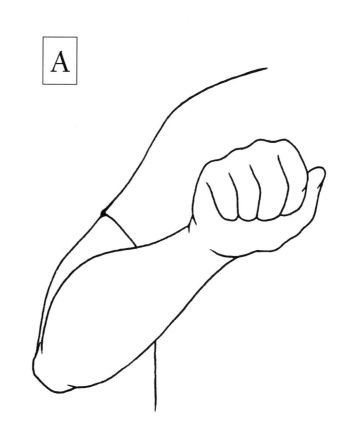

- Make a fist, keeping the thumb outside.
- Bend your wrist forward, without forcing, as far as it will go.

B

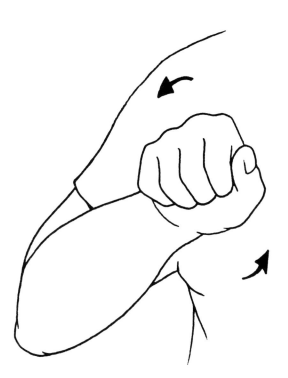

Hint: Be gentle to overworked muscles and tendons. Practice these stretches slowly and thoughtfully. See pages 13 - 16 for more information.

- Rotate your wrist in the widest circle possible.

- Allow fifteen to twenty seconds to complete one circle.

- Complete two circles in one direction, then repeat in the other direction.

WRISTS

EXERCISE 3

- Lengthens tissues on the inside of the forearm and wrist
- Improves wrist flexibility

Hint: Try closing your eyes as you perform this stretch. It will help you feel the subtleties of the Stretch Point - a very important part of this exercise.

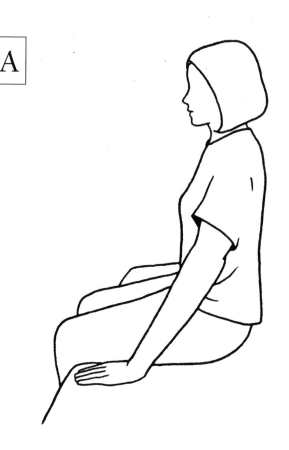

A

- Sit up straight and place your hands palm down on the seat beside you. Your hands should be several inches in front of your hips.
- This position creates a stretch point for many people with Carpal Tunnel Syndrome. Be sure to wait for the release before continuing.

CONQUERING CARPAL TUNNEL SYNDROME

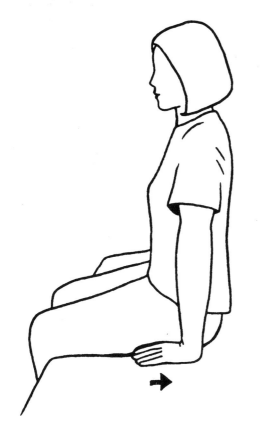

B

EXERCISE 3

Hint: Do this exercise with the arms straight, but not locked. If your arms are too short for your hands to comfortably reach the surface of the seat, place a folded towel next to your hips. This will provide you with a raised surface on which to rest your hands for this exercise. If your arms are too long, sit on a pillow. This will raise your hips and allow your arms and hands to extend to the surface of the seat.

- Slide your hands in one inch increments back toward your hips.

- Pause at each stretch point and wait for the release.

- Do not continue beyond the position illustrated.

WRISTS

. . . .

EXERCISE 4

- Excellent stretch for the

    entire forearm

- Helps restore wrist flexibility

Have you read "Self-Care Success" yet?
You can find it beginning on page 1.

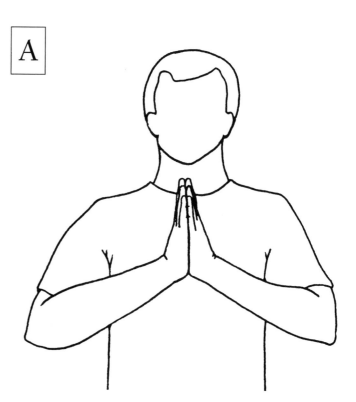

A

- Put your hands together in the traditional praying position, palms flat, fingers relaxed.
- Press the heels of your palms together firmly.
- Allow your elbows to come away from the sides of your body.

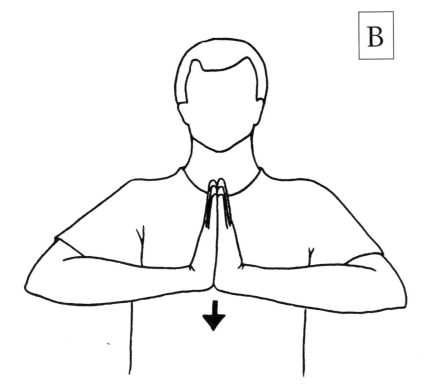

B

EXERCISE 4

Hint: This exercise works best when both wrists have the same range of motion. If you find that you can stretch one wrist farther than the other when doing this exercise, first try Exercises 7 and 8 in the Wrist section to bring balance to the flexibility of your wrists. Return to this exercise when your wrist flexibility is more consistent.

- Gently press down on the heels of your palms until you feel a stretch point. Wait for the release.

- Keep your fingers relaxed and your shoulders down.

- Continue to press down and wait for the release at each stretch point.

- Go to the next step only when both wrists and elbows are in a line, parallel to the floor.

WRISTS

EXERCISE 4

Hint: You can make this stretch easier by interlacing your fingers as you repeat all four steps of the exercise. Gradually work up to the straight finger position.

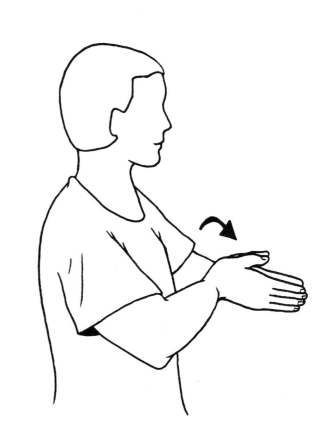

C

- Keeping the heels of your palms firmly pressed together, rotate your hands outward so your fingers point away from your body.

- Pause at each stretch point and wait for the release.

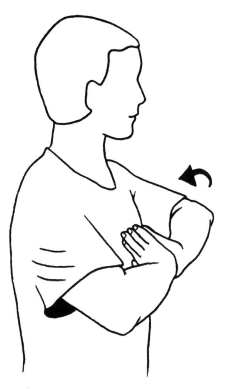

D

EXERCISE 4

Another Hint: Try this exercise as you lie on your back in bed.

Tingling and numbness occur when nerves are pinched or constricted. In cases of Carpal Tunnel Syndrome or other repetitive strain injuries of the upper body the most common sites for this type of interference are the soft tissues of the neck, front of the shoulder, elbow, and carpal tunnel of the wrist. Gentle stretching in these areas can restore restricted tissues to their normal loose and fluid state, eliminating a major source of numbness and tingling.

- Rotate your hands in the opposite direction so your fingers point toward your chest.
- Keep the heels of your palms pressed firmly together and your fingers relaxed.
- Pause at each stretch point and wait for the release.

WRISTS

EXERCISE 5

- Helps lengthen finger tendons

- Great stretch for the palm

- Lengthens forearm tissues from the elbow through the little finger

- Helps stretch tissues that may be responsible for numbness and tingling in the ring and little fingers

A

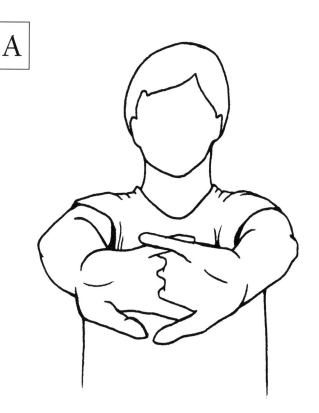

- Lace your fingers together.
- Turn your hands so your palms face outward and your elbows are straight.
- This is a strong stretch for the finger tendons. Do not go on to the next step until you can do this step without discomfort.

B

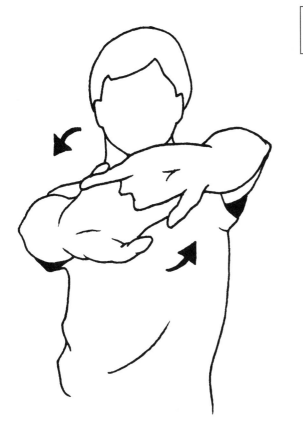

EXERCISE 5

Hint: Here's another exercise that is often easier to do while lying on your back. Extend your arms straight up toward the ceiling and proceed with the twisting motion.

- With your palms facing forward and your elbows straight, raise your left arm to create a twist.

- Wait for each stretch point and continue only after you have felt the release.

- Reverse the twist so your right arm is higher than your left. Wait for the release.

WRISTS

. . . .

EXERCISE 6

- *Stretches the back of the wrist*

- *Helps restore wrist flexibility*

- *Increases wrist range of motion*

Hint: Try pointing your fingers in different directions as they rest on your hips. It is possible to find a stretch point with nearly every direction. Experiment with finding and releasing as many new stretch points as possible. Further information about the Stretch Point begins on page 13.

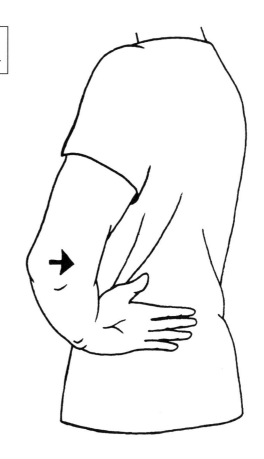

A

- Place the backs of your wrists on your hips with your elbows extended straight out to the side.

- Your fingers should be pointing back as illustrated.

- Holding your wrists and hands in place, move your elbows toward the back of your body. This will create a deeper bend in the wrist.

- This exercise works best when you keep your fingers as relaxed as possible.

BODY AWARENESS

The Flexibility of the Wrists

In order to maintain the natural strength, fluidity, and gracefulness of the hands, it is important to pay attention to the condition of the wrists. The flexibility of your wrists is essential to restoring your hands to their normal, pain-free state. Try these wrist awareness exercises to begin noticing how you are using or holding your wrists on a daily basis:

1. Hold your wrists still and walk around for a few minutes. How does wrist rigidity affect the movement of your arms? How is your breathing affected? How do your shoulders feel? Does rigidity in your wrists cause an increase or decrease in discomfort in your hands or arms?

2. Notice what you do with your wrists when you are writing. Do you freely move your wrists or do you hold them tight and still?

3. Shake hands with someone. Do you lock your wrists? Try gripping with your fingers only and allow your wrist to relax while you shake hands. Notice how this makes the handshake feel more warm and welcoming.

Joints are a common site of muscular tension in the body. Over time, we become accustomed to holding parts of our bodies still, which almost always affects the joints. Stillness causes the tissue that crosses the joints to become hard and inflexible. It is these changes that have built up over a lifetime that reduce the overall suppleness and comfort of our movements. As you continue to discover how you use your body, pay careful attention to your joints, how you hold them in stillness and how you release them into full mobility.

WRISTS

EXERCISE 7

- *Stretches the inside of the wrist*
- *Stretches the base of the thumb*
- *Lengthens muscles on the inside of the forearm*

Hint: You can vary this exercise by placing your hands on your hips with your fingertips pointing straight down. Pointing in other directions can help you find new stretch points.* Experiment to find ones that best suit your needs.

* See "What is the Stretch Point" beginning on page 13.

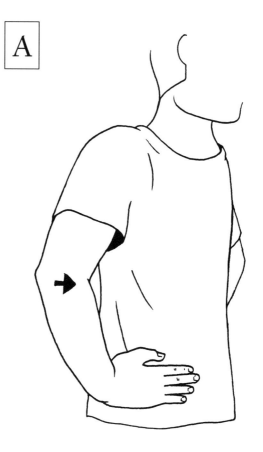

A

- Place your hands on your hips with your fingers pointing straight forward.
- Slowly roll your elbows forward to create a deeper bend in the wrists.
- Stop at each stretch point and wait for the release.
- If this position is too difficult to do without discomfort, try pointing your fingers in a slightly downward direction.

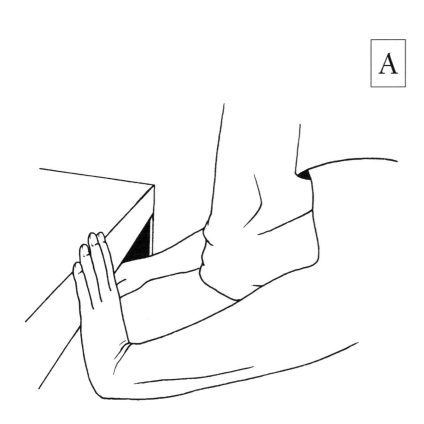

A

- *Stretches finger muscles and*

  tendons

- *Helps improve forearm*

  strength

Hint: Here's an easy stretch you can
do at your desk!

- Press your fingers against the edge of your desk,

  allowing your wrists to bend until you reach

  the first stretch point.

- Wait for the release.

- You can create a variation of this exercise by

  performing it with your fingers spread apart.

WRISTS

. . . .

EXERCISE 9

- *Stretches wrist and fingers*

- *Stretches deep muscles of the hand*

- *Lengthens muscles of the forearm*

Hint: Try this exercise two ways. First, perform it with your elbow bent. Next, try the exercise with your elbow straight. What difference do you feel?

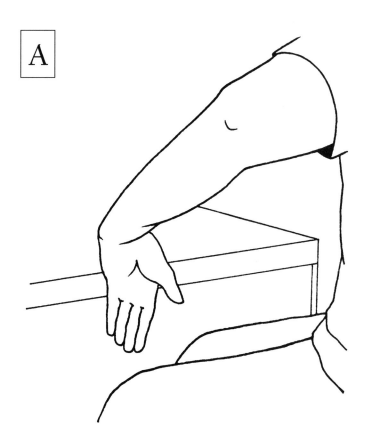

A

- Bend your wrist palmward and press the back of your wrist against the edge of a table or desk.

- Hold this position until you feel the release of the stretch point.

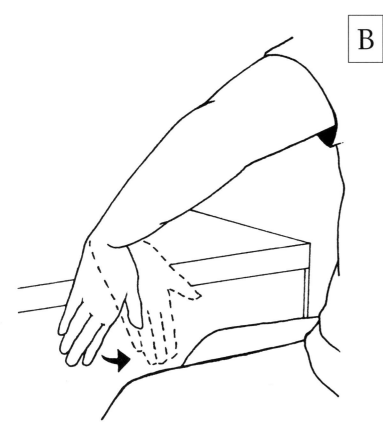

B

- Maintaining the same bend in your wrist, rotate your hand so your fingertips point toward the 7 o'clock position.

- Hold this position until a release occurs.

- Still holding the same bend in your wrist, rotate your hand so your fingertips point to the 5 o'clock position.

- Hold this position until a release occurs.

There are hundreds of ways to create stretches for the tight tissues of your body. This exercise illustrates a way to use desks or tables (you can even try this against the wall) to create stretches to relieve or prevent Carpal Tunnel Syndrome. Try to create your own unique ways to fit stretches into your day.

EXERCISE 10

- *Stretches the thumb, index and middle fingers*
- *Creates a rotary stretch for the forearm*

The Stretch Point is the most important concept to understand to get the most healing with this program. Turn to page 13 to learn about the Stretch Point.

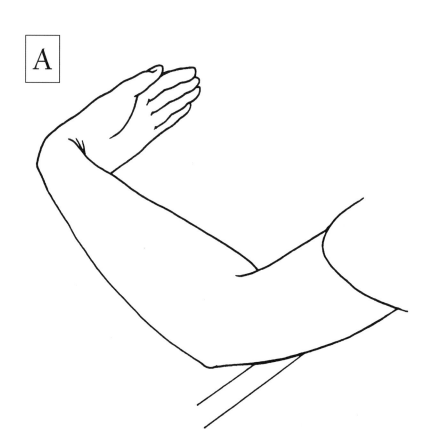

A

- Bend your wrist at a right angle, little finger on the bottom.
- Imagine that your little finger is glued to the table, preventing it from moving.

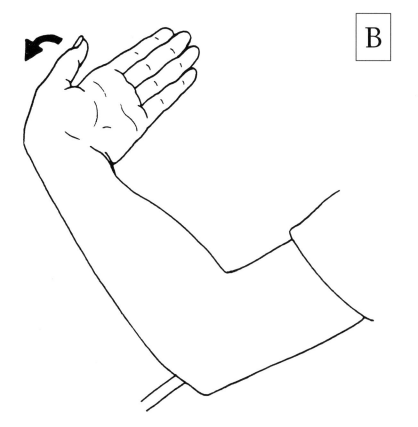

B

EXERCISE 10

Hint: For an advanced version of this exercise, try closing your fingers and thumb in a loose fist as you perform the stretch.

- Press the back of your wrist away from your body causing the back of your hand to begin rolling in the direction of your thumb.

- This exercise creates a bend and twist in the wrist at the same time.

- Pause at the stretch point and wait for the release.

NOTES

FINGERS

Fingers are amazing structures designed for strength, fluidity, and gracefulness. Surprisingly, they accomplish movement with very little muscle tissue in the fingers themselves.

The soft tissue structure of the fingers is composed mostly of connective tissue in the form of tendons. The muscles that create movements generally are located in the forearms.

Because of this unique structural feature, it is best to include several forearm stretches in your routine when trying to relieve finger tension and weakness.

FINGERS

· · · · · · · · · · · · · · · · · · · ·

EXERCISE 1

- Excellent overall stretch for the hand

- Loosens deep muscles of the palm

- Releases tight hand tissues

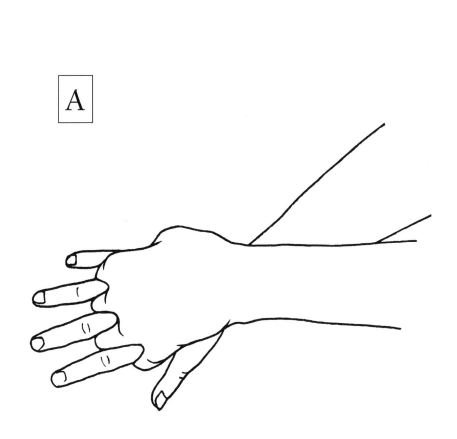

A

- Hold your right hand out in front of your body, palm down and fingers spread.

- Place your left hand on top of the right, lacing the fingers of your left hand between those of your right hand.

- Keep your left hand firmly in place.

B

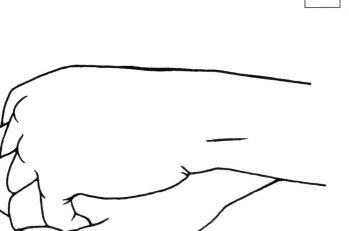

Hint: This is a wonderful exercise for relieving tension and discomfort in the palm and through the wrist. Easy to do any time of the day, it is recommended for keyboard operators and anyone doing tasks requiring a firm grip or fine, precise finger movements.

- Begin slowly closing your right hand's fingers.

- You might experience stretch points which feel like tight skin. Pause until the stretched skin sensation softens.

- Continue until you have a completely closed fist.

- Squeeze firmly and hold for twenty seconds.

- Release your grip slowly and shake out both hands before repeating with the left hand.

FINGERS

EXERCISE 2

- Stretches the deep muscles of the hand

- Increases finger flexibility and strength

- Relieves tense and sore hands

- Helps overcome the strain of continuous gripping

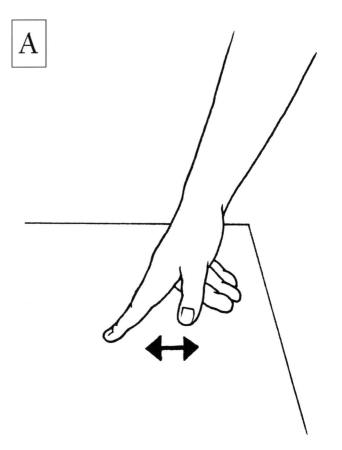

A

- Hold your hand over a table or desk so your fingers are pointing down and your palm is facing your body.

- Begin to create "splits" by allowing your index finger to slide forward while your middle finger slides back.

- Gently lower your hand, stretching the fingers apart.

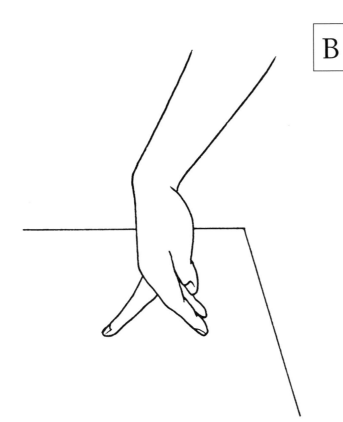

B

Important! Do not try to stretch the fingers from side to side!

Hint: You can also perform this stretch by using the fingers of one hand to stretch apart the fingers of the other hand. Take it slowly and gently.

- Reverse the stretch by allowing your middle finger to slide forward and your index finger to slide back.

- Press very gently. Never force your fingers apart.

- Repeat this sequence for all the remaining fingers on both hands.

FINGERS

Hands are such an important part of the human experience that we frequently refer to them in our language. Notice how the hands, or the function of the hands, helps convey a message. References about the human body are not limited to the hands, however. How many references about the neck, shoulders, elbows, and arms can you think of?

A bird in the hand is worth two in the bush.

HANDS OFF!

Give her a big hand!

Get a grip!

I've got to hand it to you!

What a handy tool!

HANDS UP!

Let me see a show of hands.

I've got a handle on it.

He's got a good grasp of the facts.

Can you give me a hand with this?

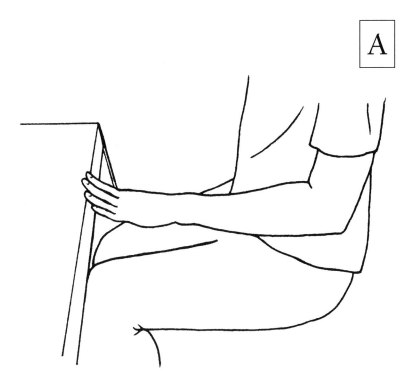

A

EXERCISE 3

- *Lengthens finger tendons*

- *Improves finger strength*

- *Reduces hand fatigue*

Hint: This is an excellent stretch for people who use a "power grip" in their work, such as when holding a power tool or the repetitive squeezing of scissors or a ticket punch. Tendons passing through the hand and into the fingers tend to become fatigued, short, and sore. This exercise helps isolate this area of the hand so that tendons can be restored to their normal length.

- While keeping your wrist straight, press your fingertips against the edge of a desk or table.

- Your fingers should bend at the joint where your fingers join your palm.

- You can create a variation by spreading your fingers apart as you press them on the edge of the table.

FINGERS

· · · · · · · · · · · · · · · · ·

EXERCISE 4

- *Stretches muscles from the fingertips through the forearms*
- *Enhances finger flexibility and strength*

Hint: Once you have achieved a more normal condition of your tendons, it is possible to maintain their good condition easily. Simply fit this exercise into your day whenever possible. Try it while you are on the phone, at a meeting, or waiting for the light to turn green at an intersection. Always remain conscious of the sensations in your hands as you stretch.

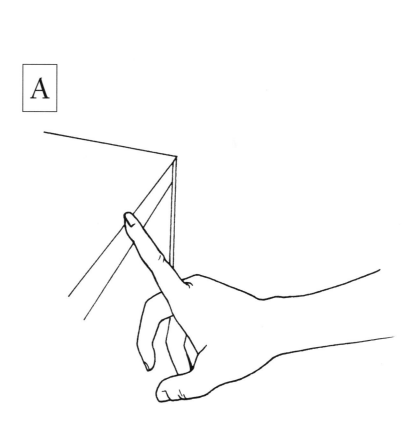

A

- Press your index finger against the edge of a table or desk, keeping your wrist straight.
- Slowly ease into the stretch point and hold the position until you feel a release.
- Keep your other fingers relaxed as you do this stretch.
- Repeat this sequence for each finger.
- Do not stretch the thumb in this fashion.

CONQUERING CARPAL TUNNEL SYNDROME

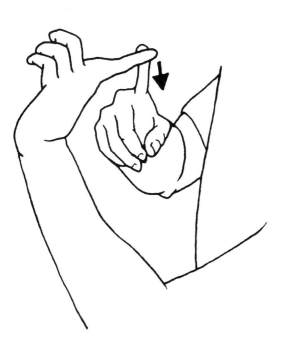

A

EXERCISE 5

- Creates maximum stretch of finger muscles through the palm
- Helps restore fine coordination of the hands
- Enhances finger strength

Hint: As an advanced exercise, continue holding each finger down after the stretch point has released. Wiggle the remaining fingers as slowly and widely as possible, being careful not to strain any of the stretching muscles. Be attentive to the sensations you are feeling if you try this advanced version of the exercise.

- Prop your left elbow on a desk or tabletop.
- Allowing your wrist to bend, pull the left index finger back until you feel a slight drag on the movement of your finger.
- Pause in this position and allow the stretch point to develop and then fully release.
- Be careful not to overstretch with this exercise.
- Repeat this sequence with the remaining fingers on both hands.

FINGERS

· · · · · · · · · · · · · · · · · · ·

It's really fun and interesting to observe the movement patterns of other people. Spend some time watching various people use their fingers. Great times to do this might include when they are lifting a coffee cup, counting money, holding a purse, carrying a child, fingering their hair, picking up a delicate object, or lifting a heavy item. Can you detect tension, relaxation, nervousness, ease, strength, or weakness with their finger movements?

BODY AWARENESS

The Unique Mobility of the Fingers

The fingers are capable of great strength as well as exquisitely fine movement. In the process of living, however, we often begin to limit the kinds of movements we ask our fingers to perform.

The health of the muscles and tendons controlling your fingers depends on the freedom and flexibility of these tissues. Try these fun finger movement patterns:

Hold your hand in front of your body, fingers straight.
1. One finger at a time, slowly curl each finger down, touching your fingertip to the palm. Return to the starting position and repeat with the next finger.

2. Beginning with the index finger, curl your fingers palmward in a wave-like fashion, ending with all fingers touching the palm. Reverse back to the starting position, again moving in a wave-like fashion. Repeat, starting with the little finger.

3. Bend the index and middle finger at the same time, then the index and the ring finger, then the index and little finger. Repeat this pattern with new combinations of fingers.

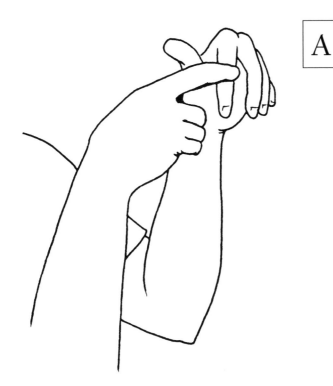

A

- *Enhances wrist and finger flexibility*
- *Promotes fluid movement of the fingers*

Hint: After you feel each release, remain in position with your finger held down. Wiggle the remaining fingers as slowly and widely as possible.

- With your left elbow propped on a tabletop, bend your hand forward at the wrist.
- Gently press your left finger down between the first and second joints.
- Press very lightly and stop when the movement of your finger "drags." This is the stretch point.
- Hold for ten seconds or until you feel the release.
- Repeat for the remaining fingers.

NOTES

THUMBS

The thumbs are an essential component of the hand. Many hand activities are difficult or impossible...without the use of the thumbs.

The muscle tissue of the thumbs often weakens or atrophies due to Carpal Tunnel Syndrome. Working slowly and carefully, you can use the exercises in this section to help strengthen the thumbs and restore them to full function.

EXERCISE 1

- *Relieves soreness and tension in the thumb*
- *Helps restore full range of motion to the thumb*
- *Helps relieve tension in the palm*

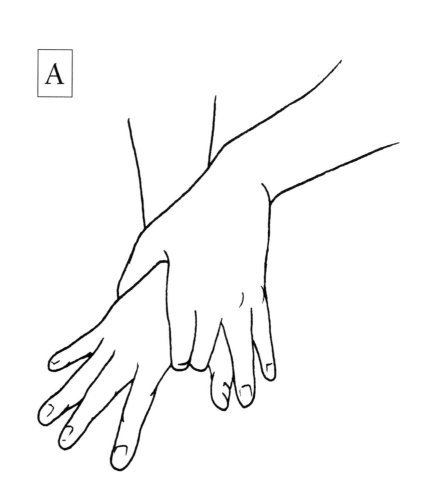

A

- Hold your right hand in front of your body, fingers spread wide apart.
- Place the first and second fingers of your left hand in the space between the thumb and forefinger of your right hand.
- Holding this position, firmly press with the left hand.

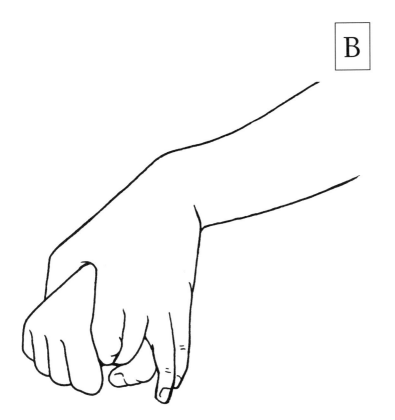

B

Exercise 1

The fleshy area between the thumb and forefinger contains an acupuncture point called "Hoku." Pressure in this area may have two-fold benefits: first, muscular tightness in the area may be released and second, the powerful balancing effect of the Hoku point may help relieve numbness in the fingers.

- Slowly close your right hand until you have a tightly closed fist.
- Hold this position for fifteen to twenty seconds.
- Release your grip and shake out both hands thoroughly.
- Reverse and repeat for the other hand.

THUMBS

. . . .

EXERCISE 2

- Reduces tension in the thumb

- Increases thumb range of

  motion

- Helps relieve tension in the

  palm

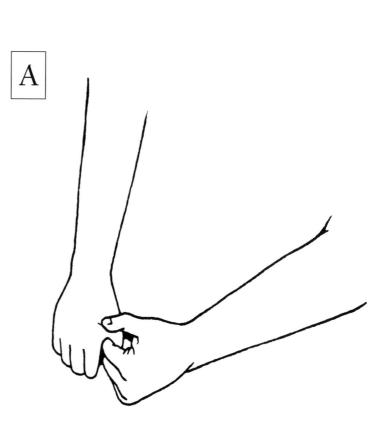

A

- Grasp the flesh between the thumb and forefinger

  of your right hand with the thumb and

  forefinger of your left hand.

- Gently squeeze this tissue while slowly closing

  your fingers and thumb.

- Hold this position for five to ten seconds.

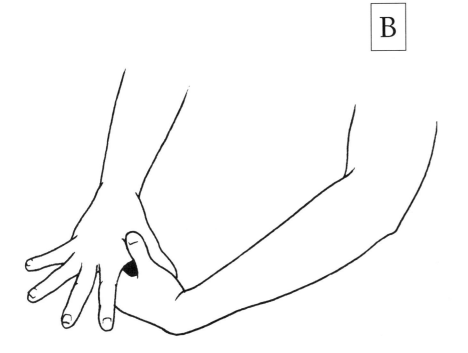

B

EXERCISE 2

Very often in Carpal Tunnel Syndrome, the muscles between the thumb and forefinger become very short and tight, pulling the base of the thumb closer to the forefinger. To maintain maximum thumb strength and flexibility, it is important to keep this area loose and open. Try this exercise to achieve this powerful effect.

- While continuing to squeeze the fleshy tissue, slowly open the fingers and thumb of your right hand until they are spread apart.
- Hold this position for five seconds.
- Reverse and repeat for the left hand.

THUMBS

· ·

EXERCISE 3

- *Stretches thumb muscles at the back of the hand*
- *Increases range of motion in the thumb*

Hint: The more slowly and softly you perform this stretch, the faster you will achieve positive results.

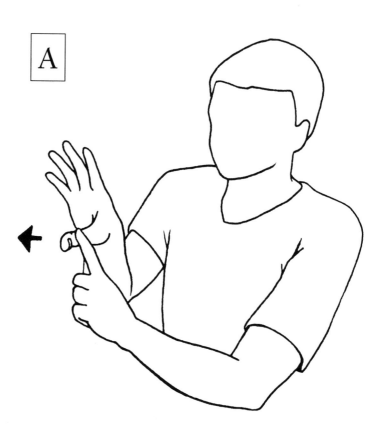

A

- With your hand held in front of your body, wrist straight, gently pull your thumb straight in front of your palm.
- Hold the stretch point until you feel a release.

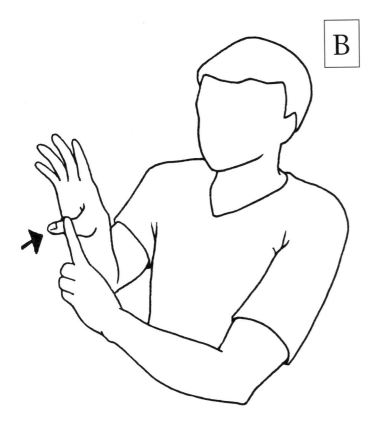

B

EXERCISE 3

Hint: For an advanced version of this exercise, try bending your thumb as you press it palmward. You can also flex your wrist sideways in the direction of the little finger. This creates a strong stretch for the thumb and should not be attempted until you can perform Exercise 3, steps A and B, with no discomfort.

- Gently pull your thumb toward the center of your palm. Keep your thumb straight.
- Hold the stretch point until you feel a release.

THUMBS

EXERCISE 4

- *Releases tension at the base of the thumb*

- *Stretches deep muscles of the thumb (palm-side)*

Your thumbs work very hard for you. Treat them gently as you encourage them to heal.

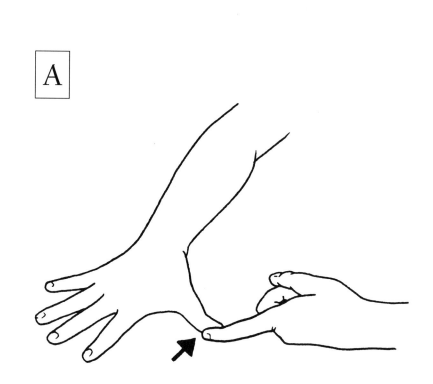

A

- Place your hand flat on a table, wrist straight.

- Gently pull the thumb away from the forefinger, creating as much distance between them as possible.

- Your other fingers should remain relaxed.

- Pause at the stretch point and wait for the release.

B

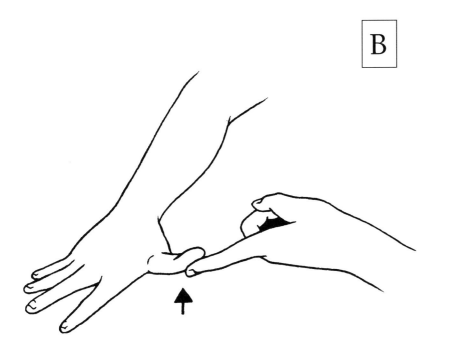

EXERCISE 4

Hint: The more softly you stretch the thumbs, the better and more effective the release.

- Keeping all other parts of your hand and arm relaxed, gently lift your thumb upward.
- Never lift more than two inches.
- Hold the stretch point until you feel the release.

EXERCISE 5

- *Stretches thumb muscles near the wrist*

- *Increases thumb flexibility and range of motion*

- *Stretches wrist tissue at the base of the thumb*

Have you read the section describing the Stretch Point? It is essential that you understand the concept of the Stretch Point in order to have the greatest success with this exercise. Please refer to pages 13 - 16 for full instruction.

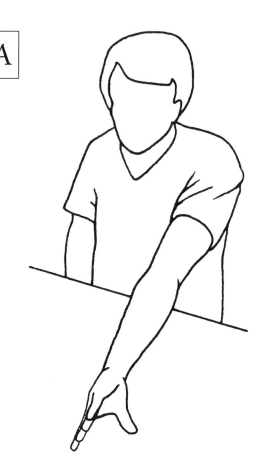

A

- Extend your arm straight in front of you on a table.

- Turn your wrist and tuck your thumb under your hand.

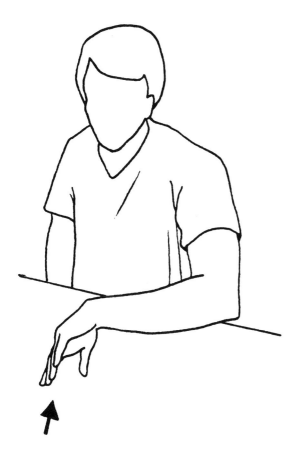

B

Hint: The thumbs are particularly sensitive areas of the hands. Always take special care to avoid overstretching. Remain aware of the sensations in your thumbs as you stretch them.

- Keeping your thumb tucked under, and with the shoulders level, begin to draw the back of your wrist toward the center of your body.

- Pause at the stretch point and wait for the release.

EXERCISE 6

- *Stretches deep thumb muscles connecting to the palm*
- *Helps keep the thumb joint flexible*
- *Mobilizes the thumb joint at the wrist*

Hint: The thumbs are particularly sensitive to overstretching. Proceed slowly and gently with this exercise.

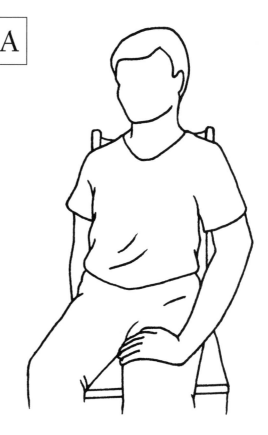

A

- Place your left hand on your left thigh with your fingers and thumb pointing toward the inside of your leg.
- Bend your elbow out to the side.
- Keep your fingers relaxed.
- Your wrist should be comfortably bent.

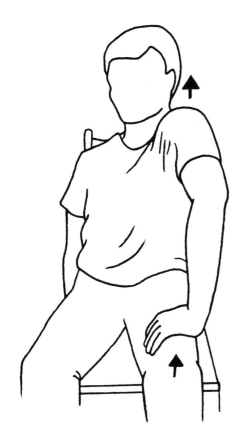

B

EXERCISE 6

The Flexor Retinaculum is a ligament which spans from the base of the thumb to the base of the little finger. This ligament helps form the carpal tunnel at the wrist. This exercise may help decompress the carpal tunnel by lengthening the Flexor Retinaculum.

- Slowly begin to shrug your left shoulder. This will cause your elbow to straighten.

- Allow the outside of your palm to roll up and away from the surface of your leg. The base of your thumb will be pressed into your leg.

- Pause at the stretch point and wait for the release.

- Be very gentle with this exercise!

THUMBS

· · · · · · · · · · · · · · · · · · ·

EXERCISE 7

- Restores fluid movement to thumb muscles as they pass through the wrist

- Helps restore the wrist to full range of motion

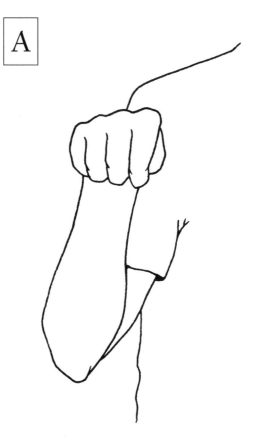

A

- Place your thumb inside your closed fist.
- Slowly rotate your fist in the widest circle possible.
- Take fifteen to twenty seconds to complete one circle.
- Do two circles, first in one direction, then in the other.
- Repeat with the other hand.

· · · · · · · · · · · · · · · · · ·

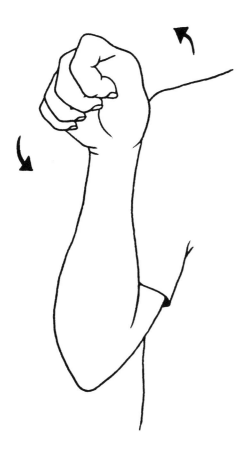

B

EXERCISE 7

Hint: While performing this stretch, take the time to pause each time you feel a stretch point, then wait for it to release, as your wrist goes around the circle. Done slowly, you will feel stretches that extend into your forearm. This will help increase the range of motion of your wrist and forearm as well as the thumb.

- For an effective stretch of the tissues of the thumb, pause when your hand tilts toward your little finger.

- Be very careful not to overstretch the small and delicate tissues of the thumb.

BUTLER RSI SOLUTIONS

Butler RSI Solutions, located in Berwyn, Pennsylvania, is an organization developed by Sharon J. Butler in 1992. Dedicated to the elimination of repetitive strain injuries of the upper body, various educational and treatment programs are offered for the individual, the corporate client, and the healthcare professional.

The key to the reduction and elimination of repetitive strain injuries is education and body conditioning. When an individual understands how injuries occur, and has been trained in techniques that can prevent or reduce those injuries, then that individual becomes an advocate on behalf of his or her own health.

Butler RSI Solutions offers several workshops, ergonomic evaluation, and custom designed exercise programs to meet the injury prevention needs of the corporate client as well as the individual. For those already experiencing a repetitive strain injury, a series of four 1 hour sessions of myofascial release and customized exercise instruction are available. The result is significant relief of symptoms as well as a comprehensive body conditioning program designed to prevent the recurrence of symptoms in the future.

Comprehensive training programs for the healthcare professional are offered once or twice per year. Training includes myofascial anatomy and physiology, myofascial release techniques for the relief of repetitive strain injury symptoms, structural evaluation, ergonomic assessment, and body conditioning program development.

Inquiries about the programs and services offered by Butler RSI Solutions are welcomed. Please direct your questions to:

Butler RSI Solutions
1273 Lancaster Avenue
Berwyn, PA 19312-1244
610-889-9683
610-889-9857 (FAX)

RESURCES

SUGGESTED READING

BODYWISE, by Joseph Heller and William A. Henkin, Wingbow Press, Oakland, CA, © 1986 & 1991.

JOB'S BODY: A Handbook for Bodywork, by Deane Juhan, Station Hill Press,Inc., Barrytown, NY, © 1987.

ROLFING, by Dr. Ida P. Rolf, PhD., Healing Arts Press, Rochester, VT, © 1977 by Dr. Ida P. Rolf and © 1989 by Alan Demmerle.

HELLERWORK

Hellerwork is a powerful system of somatic education and structural body-work which is based on the inseparability of body, mind and spirit. Hellerwork makes the connection between movement, body alignment and personal aware-ness and is based on the assumption that every person is innately healthy.

To find a Certified Hellerwork Practitioner in your area, contact:

Hellerwork International
406 Berry Street
Mount Shasta, CA 96067
1-800-392-3900
FAX: 916-926-6839

INDEX

· ·

INDEX

Some Other New Harbinger Self-Help Titles

The Self-Esteem Companion, $10.95
The Gay and Lesbian Self-Esteem Book, $13.95
Making the Big Move, $13.95
How to Survive and Thrive in an Empty Nest, $13.95
Living Well with a Hidden Disability, $15.95
Overcoming Repetitive Motion Injuries the Rossiter Way, $15.95
What to Tell the Kids About Your Divorce, $13.95
The Divorce Book, Second Edition, $15.95
Claiming Your Creative Self: True Stories from the Everyday Lives of Women, $15.95
Six Keys to Creating the Life You Desire, $19.95
Taking Control of TMJ, $13.95
What You Need to Know About Alzheimer's, $15.95
Winning Against Relapse: A Workbook of Action Plans for Recurring Health and Emotional Problems, $14.95
Facing 30: Women Talk About Constructing a Real Life and Other Scary Rites of Passage, $12.95
The Worry Control Workbook, $15.95
Wanting What You Have: A Self-Discovery Workbook, $18.95
When Perfect Isn't Good Enough: Strategies for Coping with Perfectionism, $13.95
Earning Your Own Respect: A Handbook of Personal Responsibility, $12.95
High on Stress: A Woman's Guide to Optimizing the Stress in Her Life, $13.95
Infidelity: A Survival Guide, $13.95
Stop Walking on Eggshells, $14.95
Consumer's Guide to Psychiatric Drugs, $16.95
The Fibromyalgia Advocate: Getting the Support You Need to Cope with Fibromyalgia and Myofascial Pain, $18.95
Healing Fear: New Approaches to Overcoming Anxiety, $16.95
Working Anger: Preventing and Resolving Conflict on the Job, $12.95
Sex Smart: How Your Childhood Shaped Your Sexual Life and What to Do About It, $14.95
You Can Free Yourself From Alcohol & Drugs, $13.95
Amongst Ourselves: A Self-Help Guide to Living with Dissociative Identity Disorder, $14.95
Healthy Living with Diabetes, $13.95
Dr. Carl Robinson's Basic Baby Care, $10.95
Better Boundries: Owning and Treasuring Your Life, $13.95
Goodbye Good Girl, $12.95
Fibromyalgia & Chronic Myofascial Pain Syndrome, $19.95
The Depression Workbook: Living With Depression and Manic Depression, $17.95
Self-Esteem, Second Edition, $13.95
Angry All the Time: An Emergency Guide to Anger Control, $12.95
When Anger Hurts, $13.95
Perimenopause, $16.95
The Relaxation & Stress Reduction Workbook, Fourth Edition, $17.95
The Anxiety & Phobia Workbook, Second Edition, $18.95
I Can't Get Over It, A Handbook for Trauma Survivors, Second Edition, $16.95
Messages: The Communication Skills Workbook, Second Edition, $15.95
Thoughts & Feelings, Second Edition, $18.95
Depression: How It Happens, How It's Healed, $14.95
The Deadly Diet, Second Edition, $14.95
The Power of Two, $15.95
Living Without Depression & Manic Depression: A Workbook for Maintaining Mood Stability, $18.95
Couple Skills: Making Your Relationship Work, $14.95
Hypnosis for Change: A Manual of Proven Techniques, Third Edition, $15.95
Letting Go of Anger: The 10 Most Common Anger Styles and What to Do About Them, $12.95
Infidelity: A Survival Guide, $13.95
When Anger Hurts Your Kids, $12.95
Don't Take It Personally, $12.95
The Addiction Workbook, $17.95
It's Not OK Anymore, $13.95
Beyond Grief: A Guide for Recovering from the Death of a Loved One, $14.95
The Chemotherapy & Radiation Survival Guide, Second Edition, $14.95
An End to Panic: Breakthrough Techniques for Overcoming Panic Disorder, Second Edition, $18.95
Dying of Embarrassment: Help for Social Anxiety and Social Phobia, $13.95
The Endometriosis Survival Guide, $13.95
Grief's Courageous Journey, $12.95
Flying Without Fear, $13.95
Stepfamily Realities, $14.95
Coping With Schizophrenia: A Guide For Families, $15.95
Conquering Carpal Tunnel Syndrome and Other Repetitive Strain Injuries, $17.95
The Three Minute Meditator, Third Edition, $13.95
The Chronic Pain Control Workbook, Second Edition, $17.95
The Power of Focusing, $12.95
Living Without Procrastination, $12.95
Kid Cooperation: How to Stop Yelling, Nagging & Pleading and Get Kids to Cooperate, $13.95

Call **toll free, 1-800-748-6273,** or log on to our online bookstore at **www.newharbinger.com** to order. Have your Visa or Mastercard number ready. Or send a check for the titles you want to New Harbinger Publications, Inc., 5674 Shattuck Ave., Oakland, CA 94609. Include $3.80 for the first book and 75¢ for each additional book, to cover shipping and handling. (California residents please include appropriate sales tax.) Allow two to five weeks for delivery.

Prices subject to change without notice.